A Well Model Approach
to Care of the Dying Client

A Well Model Approach to Care of the Dying Client

Arlene McGrory, R.N., M.S.

Instructor
University of Lowell
Massachusetts

McGraw-Hill Book Company

New York   St. Louis   San Francisco   Auckland   Bogotá
Düsseldorf   Johannesburg   London   Madrid   Mexico
Montreal   New Delhi   Panama   Paris   São Paulo   Singapore
Sydney   Tokyo   Toronto

A WELL MODEL APPROACH TO CARE OF THE DYING CLIENT

1 2 3 4 5 6 7 8 9 0 DODO 7 8 3 2 1 0 9 8 7 6

This book was set in Times Roman by Creative Book Services, subsidiary of McGregor & Werner, Inc. The editor was Orville W. Haberman, Jr., and the production supervisor was Milton J. Heiberg.
R. R. Donnelley & Sons Company was printer and binder.

Library of Congress Cataloging in Publication Data

McGrory, Arlene.
    A well model approach to care of the dying client.

    Includes index.
    1. Nurse and patient. 2. Terminal care.
3. Nursing. I. Title. [DNLM: 1. Attitude to death
—Nursing texts. 2. Terminal care—Nursing texts.
3. Models, Theoretical—Nursing texts. WY152 M147w]
RT86.M25   610.73′6   78-6827
ISBN 0-07-045094-3

To Ann

*I never would have begun
the book without you.*

Contents

Preface

Another book about death and dying! Why write another book of generalizations about the dying, which often hinder one from viewing individual characteristics. We need to look at dying as the process of living with the threat of death. The person tries to adapt as best as possible. The dying person is physically ill but may be emotionally well. This book is the result of years of giving direct care to dying clients and teaching student nurses a more humanistic approach to caring for the dying client. We must learn to see the client's strengths and not just the weaknesses. Moreover, we must also be the client's advocate. For this reason I propose the well model.

Since most people die in hospitals and most nurses work in hospitals, it is appropriate that care of the dying be taught to nursing students and nurses. Until recently, care of the dying has been taught as postmortem care, but at last the process of dying is being recognized as a legitimate concern of nurses.

Nurses in any stage of professional development can use the concepts in this book. Emphasis is placed on nurses becoming more sensitive to the often conflicting personal feelings about death and the dying process. Faculty can use the book, especially Chapter 8, as a set of guidelines for adaptation to their particular program. In addition, other health care workers may find my thoughts helpful.

You will note that throughout the book the words *client* and *person* replace the traditional word *patient*. My preference for *client* is based on the perception that a client is one whose interest is represented by a professional. *Person* implies individual identity and self-determination. Unlike *patient*, which presumes that an individual is ill and is a passive recipient of treatment, a client or a person is an active and possibly well participant very much involved in this care.

Chapter 1 makes the reader aware of feelings about his or her own death. Reasons why it is important to think about dying are presented.

Chapter 2 describes obstacles that limit the care-related options of the dying client. Historically in the United States the health care system has taken away the client's self-determination and has depersonalized this care.

Chapter 3 presents the theoretical framework for a broad-based well model approach to nursing. The essential terms and concepts defined in this book are health, wellness, adaptation, stress, equilibrium, margin of equilibrium safety, sickness, and maladaptation. Seven assumptions support the well model. The well model is explained schematically by adapting Lewin's field theory. Also important in using the well model are the clear identification of mutual goals and the need for advocacy by nurses.

Chapter 4 discusses the well model as it applies to the nursing process in general. It is useful in both distributive and episodic settings. The problem-oriented record is evaluated in the light of the well model's emphasis on the client's coping abilities and strengths. The alternative strength-oriented nursing record, based on the concepts of stress, coping, and crisis for the client, is suggested.

Chapter 5 reviews the salient concepts relevant to the dying process in general, which are crisis, grief, body image, and pain. The rights of the terminally ill client are discussed, as is the role of the advocate. The well model is applied to these concepts.

Chapter 6 is devoted to the special needs and problems of acutely dying clients. Temporal environmental conditions impinge on the provision of comfort care. The frightened client must use emergency coping mechanisms to maintain equilibrium. Guidelines are presented to meet the many needs of these clients, needs for a positive body image, physical care, control over one's environment, self-esteem, grief, life review, pain relief, and spirituality. The family is also in crisis. All these concepts are related to the well model. In addition, nurses' reactions and some solutions to problems encountered in this setting are discussed.

Chapter 7 focuses on the care required by chronically dying clients. Well model concepts are used to assess the strengths and problems of these clients. Crisis can occur at many points as losses accumulate. The needs of the chronically dying are the same as those listed for the acutely dying, but because of the longer trajectory, they present different problems. In addition, problems of the elderly, who have a high incidence of chronic illness, are also examined. Well model concepts are used throughout the chapter. Also, the advantages and disadvantages of home versus institutional care are mentioned. If care is to be rendered at home, family teaching is especially important. Finally, this chapter discusses nurses' reactions to care of the chronically dying and ways in which emotional supports can be established.

Chapter 8 presents guidelines for teaching death and dying to students. The course can be integrated or separate, preferably in a multidisciplinary environment. Students need to be taught use of crisis-intervention strategies. The format of the actual course should be determined by previous experience and expressed needs of the participants, number of hours allotted to the course, availability of resources, faculty preparation, and clinical facilities available.

As a person, nurse, teacher, and student, I continue to develop my understanding of myself and my dying clients as living, breathing human beings. I hope the reader will also do this.

Finally, I would like to acknowledge with many thanks the people who supported the preparation of the book. The Ella Lyman Cabot Fund provided the finances to meet the manuscript-preparation expenses. Alyce Cocqueran and family provided me a warm, hospitable place to stay and a needed respite on my trips to New York. The photographs and constructive criticism of the manuscript are Patricia Roderick's contribution. For helpful editing suggestions I thank Ellen Pfeifer and Tobey Conlin. To all my friends and colleagues, especially Dr. Arnald Gurin, dean of the School of Social Work, Brandeis University, who were so supportive when I was discouraged I am deeply grateful. Finally, I thank my typists, Ursula Dafeldecker and Norma Panico.

Arlene McGrory

Chapter 1

Becoming Aware of Your Feelings

When is the best time to think about dying? It is not a few moments before death. That time should be spent reaping the mental rewards of a completed life. Thinking about death and dying while well may motivate one to place more value on the quality of life. More important, for the healthy person, time remains to improve capacity for living. For the chronically ill person, a shortened life span and a diminished quality of life provide the opportunity to reflect on maximizing the quality of living. Creative effort can lead to fuller utilization of remaining abilities; for instance, wheelchair basketball is a popular activity for paraplegic clients.

The initial impetus for thinking about death usually occurs during childhood. As early as 3 to 8 years of age, confrontation, sometimes indirect, with death is forced on one when a relative, a friend, or even a pet dies. The effect of this first death depends on the age-related ability to understand and the type of assistance, if any, received. Although total comprehension of the mystery of death may be impossible, its reality henceforth does exist. The child spends some time, with or without assistance, thinking about the personal implications of death. Attempts of parents to conceal death from a child therefore are usually unsuccessful.

Children frequently grow up having learned that discussing death, like sex, is taboo. They continue to have unexpressed feelings and questions about death as they mature into adulthood.

Therefore, it is necessary to ask and attempt to answer two basic questions: Why think about dying? Who is dying? There is no one right answer. Each person's sense of reality is going to affect his or her view of death, as it affects the view of life.

WHY THINK ABOUT DYING?

Healthy people often feel that their death is far removed from them, which is a comfort. Why should they think about death? Dying is an integral part of living. It is virtually impossible to shield oneself from death. Family members and close friends die.

Beyond our personally significant relationships, our larger environment represents death in frequently sensationalistic and bizarre terms, although impersonally. War and starvation are reported in statistical figures while at the same time the dying individual is a human interest story to the media.

Other deathlike situations arise to stimulate thoughts about death. Although not physical deaths, the separations of people by divorce, by political exile, or by imprisonment elicit a kind of grieving. The divorced lament the end of a relationship, the exiled mourn the loss of a homeland, and the imprisoned suffer restraints on personal freedom.

There are intangible benefits in considering death's consequences. The struggle to find meaning from life's end may be the impetus for the setting of realistic goals for living. Reflection on one's current life-style can result in improving the quality of one's life by reordering one's priorities.

The person who sees in death the loss of loved ones may make an extra effort to repair broken or strained relationships·or may value close relationships even more. In facing a finite, temporal life some people find a stronger need for spiritual relationships. Spirituality can bring solace, peace, and, for some people, the answer to the "why" of suffering, pain, and death. For the well person time and energy remain to make the most of the remaining life.

Regardless of the degree of wellness, thoughts of death affect every person's innermost feelings. Identification and examination of feelings, attitudes, and values leads to greater insight when facing a dying situation. Although this is true for both the lay person and the professional, recognition and understanding of feelings, attitudes, values, and beliefs is especially significant for nurses. Nurses react to death as individuals before they react as professionals with job titles and responsibilities. Their personal feelings influence the kind of care given.

Before entering the client's realm, it is necessary for nurses to identify their feelings about dying and specifically about their own deaths. Although total comprehension may be impossible, each attempt at reflection provides heightened self-awareness. This clarity and understanding of one's feelings

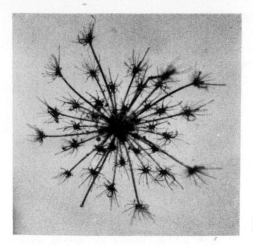

Figure 1-1 To surrender life to its natural process is to allow its ultimate serenity and fulfillment.

paves the way to a fuller understanding of the client's reaction to the dying process.

Because nurses are frequently involved in situations associated with prolongation of life, it is mandatory for the sake of their clients that they reflect on their feelings relative to living and dying. What is acceptable living as well as acceptable dying must be clarified by each individual nurse and client. Respect for a client's values must be considered. No one can decide what is acceptable living for another.

These, then, are some of the reasons one needs to think about dying.

WHO IS DYING?

Are you dying? The answer to this question is yes. At any moment, every living thing in the process of completing a life span is dying. Propelled by natural life cycles, some living substances are closer to death than others. Although the worm, tree, and human being may be dying simultaneously, the death of the human being is especially significant. The human capacity to think and reason allows us to consider the meaning of life and death. Respect for life and its inherent dignity can be the impetus for considering the quality of the process of living. This process continues until life does not exist.

For nurses, respect for clients' life and dignity should be paramount. Nurses must give this respect in the context of the nurse-client interaction by permitting clients to experience choices in their living and dying care.

The following example taken from the nurse-client interaction describes how the goals of the nurse and client can be at odds. An 87-year-old widower, Mr. M., living alone in a rooming house, barely existing on his monthly Social Security check, may consider hospitalization a blessing. It may signify that at last his life is ending. Alas, the health care team and the techniques of modern medicine reverse his pulmomary edema and help his failing heart to become compensated. He is discharged on medications and a special diet, with instructions to return to a medical clinic in 2 weeks. A visiting nurse is contacted to provide appropriate teaching and support and to assure his following the prescribed medical regimen. However, a problem develops when, as before, Mr. M. refuses to allow the visiting nurse to enter his room.

One can easily imagine the consequences of Mr. M.'s actions. He does not fill his prescription for medication, does not adhere to his diet, and subsequently is readmitted during an acute episode of pulmonary edema.

Nurses react to Mr. M.'s readmission in individualized ways. Some nurses are angry because Mr. M. did not follow their instructions, others are frustrated because their teaching techniques have not been effective, and still others are sorry he did not die on the way to the hospital.

There are other possible reasons for Mr. M.'s readmission that cannot be overlooked. Mr. M. may have a hearing impairment and may not have heard the instructions. Perhaps he really was not helped to understand his diet, or no one has asked him what he wants. If he told them, would they hear and heed his request? Maybe he just wants to die.

SUMMARY

The child inevitably confronts death. Unfortunately, he or she usually is not allowed to discuss it, so in adulthood the habit of suppression remains. Today is the time to begin thinking of the implications dying has for each one of us. Whatever degree of health we possess can be used to more fully utilize the remainder of our lives.

Nurses, as people, react to death personally before they react to death professionally. This personal reaction influences the care given. It is imperative that nurses reflect on their feelings about life and death. The nurse, along with the physician, for many clients is the gatekeeper who allows or does not allow a peaceful death.

QUESTIONS FOR REFLECTION AND DISCUSSION

1-1   When was your first experience with death? How old were you?
1-2   Was this the death of an animal, a plant, or a person? If it was a person, was it a friend or a relative?
1-3   What were the circumstances of this death? What was this person's age? How old were you?
1-4   Have you ever experienced the death of a family member? If so, describe the circumstances. Were you close to this person?
1-5   What feelings do you remember experiencing immediately after this death? Weeks later? Months and years later?
1-6   Did you ever talk to anyone about this experience?
1-7   Do you feel that you have resolved this experience?

1-8 Did anyone help you work through your grief? If so, who was this person and how was he or she helpful?

1-9 Have you had subsequent experiences with death? If so, how were they similar? Different?

QUESTIONS RELATED TO CLINICAL EXPERIENCE

1-1 Have you experienced the death of a client? If so, what were the circumstances?

1-2 What were your feelings? What did you "do"?

1-3 What were the reactions of the people around you?

1-4 Did you relate this experience to your instructor? What was the response? Was it helpful to you?

1-5 Did anyone else help you resolve your feelings?

1-6 What are the most unpleasant and difficult aspects of caring for a dying client?

BIBLIOGRAPHY

Dumont, R., and Foss, D.: *The American View of Death: Acceptance or Denial*, Cambridge, Mass., Schenkman Publishing Co., 1972.

Peretz, D.: "Development, Object-Relationships, and Loss," in Schoenberg, B., et al. (eds.), *Loss and Grief: Psychological Management in Medical Practice*, New York, Columbia University Press, 1970.

Chapter 2

Choosing How to Die

Question: If you could pick the manner in which you preferred to die, what would be your choice?

Response: I'd like to die in my sleep quietly and painlessly.

This familiar response attests to the type of death a person would prefer. For most people this wish cannot be fulfilled. Most deaths occur in an illness-related situation. However, a more peaceful death can be achieved by allowing clients freedom of choice even in this sickness milieu. Where they would like to die, who will be with them, and what kind of treatment they will receive are factors over which clients should be able to exercise some choice.

The following obstacles to client choice can occur to any person seeking health care services, but dying clients are especially affected by these obstacles because of the curtain of silence that sometimes still exists in communicating with them.

FORMULAS FOR CARE

A familiar obstacle to the health care worker and to the nurse in particular is the "patient" care plans. Frequently based on the textbook picture of the

client's medical diagnosis, these plans, when utilized improperly, become formulas for care. Originally devised to help coordinate care, these plans are
beneficial only when implemented by the entire nursing staff. Initially one nurse
obtains the nursing history, writes an assessment, and plans for implementation
of care. The plans use many familiar catchall words, which become formulas
for care. How can a nurse ''give reassurance'' and ''provide emotional support''? These phrases could mean almost anything. Interpretations are as variable as the people reading the care plan. Having no real education in this area,
nurses must base their actions on intuition or on a formula from a book on
interpersonal communications.

Another obstacle exists when the nurse assumes that the written plan
presents a complete picture of the client. Since completeness is presumed, the
plan often becomes irrevocable or subject to only minor modifications. The
nurse who prepared the plan may have overlooked or misinterpreted the client's
statements, however. For any number of reasons, the client may not have
provided all needed information to the nurse. Nurses must be constantly vigilant
in using the nursing process to update and change the care plan. The team
approach can also help to validate information. Care plans, like living, should
always be in process.

There are chemistry formulas, but there are no dying formulas. People die
in their own unique manner, and nurses must adapt care plans and care to each
individual. This is not to say that nurses must be passive but, rather, that they
should actively assist clients to die in their particular fashion.

ATTITUDE OF DENIAL VERSUS ATTITUDE OF ACCEPTANCE

Many writers have sought to identify the prevailing attitudes of American
culture as a basis for understanding the issues of death and dying. The literature
is meant to reflect societal attitudes. Since the subject of death and dying is
no longer taboo, witness the proliferation of books on the subject in recent
years. The literature also affects societal attitudes. This section is not set forth
as a conclusive treatise on the entire body of literature related to the denial or
acceptance of death. Rather, the intention is to cite those attitudes that are
usually presented as all-or-nothing dictums. For example, denial is frequently
thought of as a general precept or single mental operation unifying all psychological processes related to dying. This viewpoint inhibits further inquiry into
the way our contemporary culture views dying by reinforcing limited ideas or
misconceptions.

Historically, the psychoanalytic tradition has focused on dominant themes
of avoidance, denial, and fear of death as motivating factors in each person's
life. The words *denial, avoidance*, and *fear* each have a slightly different definition, but these words are used interchangably to refer to the negation and
avoidance of unpleasant feelings, from which a person defends self by
repression.

Most of the literature supports the denial thesis, that is, that our American culture refuses to look openly at and to accept death. Such an attitude demands that if death and dying is to be discussed at all, it should be done symbolically and euphemistically. In hospitals we transport the dead to the morgue via back corridors and elevators or we close the clients' doors. The euphemism "code 99" calls the medical personnel to a resuscitation. The old, useless, and dying are put away in nursing homes to be forgotten except on holidays. Funeral directors prepare the dead body to look as if it is sleeping or, in one mourner's words, to "look better than he has in 20 years."

A more dynamic interpretation of denial is presented by Weisman. He postulates that a person who is denying death can do so only after its existence has been accepted. Denial, therefore, is not just the avoidance of unpleasant feelings, but a defense against the loss of a significant key person and a subsequent loss of self-esteem.

There are degrees of denial. *First-order denial* relates to perception of primary illness. *Second-order denial* refers to implications drawn about the consequences of the illness. *Third-order denial* refers to denial of death as ultimate extinction. At serious transition points, middle knowledge or vacillation between denial and open acceptance can occur. In effect denial expresses itself in endless variety and forms.

Some of the literature relating to this all-or-nothing dictum presents the viewpoint that American culture accepts death. Expressions of grief at a funeral are accepted and expected. Grief is generally expected to be borne in private afterwards, and a stoic countenance is expected in public, thereby affirming that death is a natural process.

Because the medical profession accepts death, millions of dollars are spent each year seeking cures for the most common causes of death in the United States, that is, heart disease and cancer. In addition, medical researchers have developed many lifesaving machines, medicines, and treatments.

In the daily activities of each individual, acceptance of the possibility of death can be seen in the widespread use of seat belts in automobiles.

Death is a constant theme in both verbal and visual media:

> Some have argued that American acccpetance of death in the entertainment media seems to have reached a point of morbid preoccupation testified to by the marked degree of violence shown on television, and in the movies, heavy sales of "horror films," and "horror comic books," and the thousands of ill-written paperback books on the horror of war and concentration camps.[1]

The point to be made is not whether the American culture accepts or denies death, but how each of us uses denial and acceptance in our daily lives. Serious personal threat—and dying is the ultimate serious personal threat for many— may require the use of denial and acceptance at different times.

---

[1]R. Dumont and D. Foss, *The American View of Death: Acceptance or Denial*, Cambridge, Mass., Schenkman Publishing Co., 1972, pp. 54–55.

Moreover, that there is a body of literature at all supporting the denial thesis leads one to believe that there are definite constraints on the way death and dying is discussed. Understanding these constraints should make one more sensitive to the needs of the dying person and the person's loved ones.

MODERN HOSPITAL AND MEDICAL PRACTICE

In earlier times people died at home. The few existing hospitals were often inaccessible to the sick person. Thus, care of the sick fell to the family. The family circle was maintained even after death, as family members prepared the body for burial, carried the coffin to the cemetery, and buried it themselves. Dying was an acknowledged part of the life cycle.

Today medical practice and hospital care have become obstacles to a peaceful death. When 70 to 80 percent of the United States population dies in hospitals, institutional philosophy and physicians' attitudes significantly affect clients' deaths. With the exception of hospitals specifically designed for the terminally ill, hospital philosophy usually embraces the concept of cure and return to maximum functioning. The Hippocratic Oath compels physicians to relieve suffering, prolong and protect life, and do no harm. Recognition of life's end is not included in these philosophies; therefore death is not an acceptable goal. A walk through a hospital corridor by any health care worker or lay person would attest to the many new therapies in general use ostensibly to cure illness but actually to prolong life. Many books have been written about the new therapies to prolong life.

Glaser and Strauss conducted extensive studies of the sociology of dying in hospitals. Not only did they find out the interaction patterns of clients, but in addition they identified many ways by which nurses reduce their own anxiety. A dying hospitalized client may be put at the end of the corridor: out of sight and out of mind. A sense of hopelessness pervades the atmosphere around the terminally ill. Little effort is made to talk to the client because personnel feel so helpless. Another example of avoidance by nurses to reduce anxiety is forgetting to answer the call light: The client who cries in pain or asks for pain medication more frequently than it is ordered may find the door of his or her room closed. A closed door reduces anxiety for personnel.

The Hospital Administration's Aura

Whether a modern steel and concrete high-rise structure or an old-fashioned wood or brick-framed building, a hospital is alien territory to everyone, clients included, except hospital personnel. Historically, hospitals developed in the Middle Ages as resting places for weary travelers. Then, before asepsis, hospitals became havens for paupers. The hospital was a place to go and die. It was safer to stay home if a person could afford to. Now hospitals are places to go to be treated, cured, and returned home.

The complex organization of today's hospital requires the coordination of several dozen departments with varying degrees of direct effect on the client.

Many problems occur with the consequent overlapping and interdependent functions of these departments because lines of responsibility become blurred. The hospital acts as a hotel, school, and laboratory and performs many more functions. The whole process focuses on treatment and care of clients.

The administrator ultimately has the responsibility for bureaucratic functions such as policy making, budgeting, and overall efficiency of the hospital. Since most hospitals are non profit organizations, enough money must be spent to provide the most efficient service considering hospital income. Efficient service is equated with the best medical care, but the best medical care is not necessarily equated with the most personalized care. Ideally, the well-being of the client is primary, but because of the many constraints on running an efficient organization, the goal of client care may be subverted and hospital self-maintenance may become the primary goal.

While the client rarely sees the administrator, the administrator's effects can be felt through the hospital hierarchy. One policy-making decision, for example, directly affecting the client is visiting hours. Clients are aware that through the desk clerk in the lobby, the nurse on duty, and the security guard, hospital policy limiting the time and number of visitors per client is executed.

On occasion, clients have opportunities to interact with administrators directly. Since time is limited, the administrator may initiate the interaction by making cursory rounds. The ineffective conversation usually proceeds along these lines:

> *Administrator*:   How are you today?
> *Client*:   Fine.
> *Administrator*:   How is your care?
> *Client*:   Fine.

If the client is not feeling fine and does not think the care is adequate, the opportunity has been lost to speak up. The reasons he or she does not do this can be many. Again the person is relinquishing independence, autonomy, and integrity. One hopes the client does not feel intimidated by the administrator. This kind of visit helps the administrator because he or she thinks it is a way of maintaining contact with clients.

Another way a client interacts with the administration is by being a Very Important Person, such as a hospital trustee. It is good public relations to visit Very Important People.

A third way a client interacts with the administration is by having a serious medicolegal problem or by threatening to sue the hospital. The client who does not sue the hospital but has very vocal complaints may be a potential legal and public relations problem. The administrator may also visit this client.

Nurses' Perceptions

When the nurse first encounters the dying person, the situation usually is confined to the sick role. The client may be hospitalized, may be being followed in the community setting or may be being treated for complications from a chronic illness. What, then, is the significance of the interaction between the nurse and client as it relates to death and dying? Individual perceptions and goals greatly influence the meaning, duration, and intensity of the interaction. Historically, the teaching of nurses has concentrated on healing, rehabilitation, and a return to maximum functioning. The concepts pertaining to living, then, are antithetical to dying. Unfortunately, in many instances, the goals of nurses and physicians still focus on the preservation of life. The quality of life is an afterthought that is considered only when the physical needs have been met. What happens when the client is not involved in planning care or given an opportunity to express feelings about that care? The "client" becomes the "patient."

A very recent trend in the education of nurses has been the inclusion of instruction relative to assisting the client to die peacefully.

It is important to note that nurses caring for the dying client are at risk. The more they care, the more vulnerable they become to experiencing some of their clients' psychic pain. Nurses can take one of two directions in caring for the dying person. The first and the more rewarding is to get involved in really caring. A nurse becomes an *active listener* by giving full attention to the person with whom he or she is communicating, hearing the words, and observing facial expressions and gestures to understand the full meaning of the communication. Using intuitive and learned professional attitudes and behaviors, nurses solve problems. Their personal characteristic of empathy helps them give compassionate care. They learn that they cannot divorce themselves from their feelings when they care for a dying person.

The second direction nurses may take is fraught with frustration. Since nurses' perceptions of the dying process also influence the care rendered, *preconceived notions* and *stereotyped attitudes*, which form *distorted perceptions*, may block communication. Active listening then cannot take place. A preconceived notion is any idea or opinion determined before it is validated with factual information. If a nurse, for example, thinks that a client denies impending death, like all Americans, because the client will not discuss it with the nurse, communication is blocked.

Other reasons for clients' reluctance to discuss their forthcoming death may be physical or interpersonal. They may be too tired to talk or unable to hear or speak adequately. The noisy, impersonal, and open environment of the intensive care unit may inhibit clients from revealing this very personal part of themselves. Perhaps previous discussions with families and friends have made the nurses' intervention unnecessary. The clients also may sense the nurses' discomfort. There are many other possible and very individual reasons why these clients may not want to talk at this time. Nurses should respect these reasons and should not label the clients resisting and nonreceptive, for if they do they will react to those clients with frustration, anger, and anxiety. These feelings may be the result of the nurses' misunderstanding of their clients' needs, the nurses' goals, and preconceived analysis.

Stereotyped attitudes categorize personal characteristics simplistically. They convey positive or negative attributes but invariably limit perception. The client, for instance, may be labeled "demanding" if he or she wants pain medication more frequently than every 4 hours. Stereotyped attitudes prevent nurses from seeing the unique characteristics and needs of each client.

Another kind of distortion can occur when a nurse's personal feelings about a particular situation overcome professional ability to deal with the situation. Some people call this "sympathy." Again an incomplete analysis of the real situation takes place. The nurse who feels very uncomfortable when caring for a client with leukemia because all male leukemics remind her of her dead father may, by her behavior and attitude, impart a sense of hopelessness to the client and family when in fact steps can be taken to improve the quality of the remaining life. On the other hand, this personal feeling may provoke caring concern or other positive responses. The attitude of hopelessness may bring premature closure to a client's situation in that the client may feel abandoned.

To have a preconceived notion, a stereotype, or another perceptual distortion is to not listen effectively and to prevent mutually satisfying nursing intervention.

Nurses' Aura

Clients have come to expect certain attitudes and behaviors from their nurses. These expectations have developed from previous experiences, from accounts of another person's previous experiences, and from historical and current fictional stereotypes. The variety of these views about nurses extends from that of the brisk, starched, cold, efficient nurse to that of the angel of mercy in white. Nevertheless, the stereotype includes the nurse as handmaiden to the physician. Sexist stereotypes are pervasive throughout the medical and nursing professions. To the public the nurse's role does not include independent practice.

The nurse is looked upon as the overworked pill pusher or bedpan giver. Some clients find the nurse more approachable than the physician in answering questions. However, other clients think any important question cannot be answered by the nurse and must be asked directly of the physician.

Nevertheless, it is nurses with whom hospitalized clients interact on a 24 hour basis. Their control over the hospital environment is acknowledged in many ways. They are the persons who can relieve pain or encourage painful exercises. They can answer or ignore literal or figurative calls for help. In a study on clients' perceptions of nurses in hospitals these comments were significant:

Fears of displeasing others were intense for patients who felt dependent on a fast response to their calls and who dreaded being alone during a sudden, unexpected crisis. Some of these patients refused to make less urgent requests, in the hope that they would secure for themselves reliable services when the "real need"

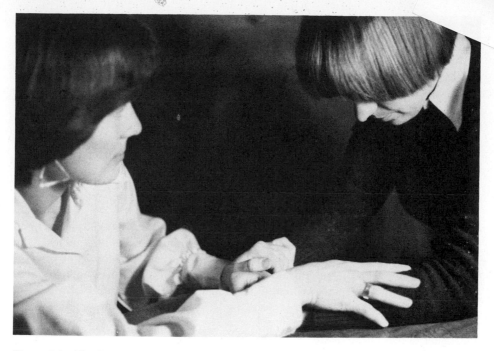

Figure 2-1   Tho degreo to which clients feel cared for and cared about is the degree to which clients feel that nurses fulfill their obligation to them.

arises. They tried, as one patient expressed it, to "save the button" in the *hope* [italics mine] that any call for a nurse would be taken seriously.[1]

In the same study both clients and nurses agreed that the essence of nursing is caring. Eighty-one percent of respondents stressed the importance of personalized care and emphasized personality attributes. Only 29 percent expected knowledge and technical skills. The clients who feel cared for and cared about are the clients who feel that nurses fulfill their obligation:

> Patients described how a slow response intensified physical discomfort and how it can trigger anger because the patient is made to feel helpless and dependent. . . . A prompt response was also important because it communicated . . . that the nurse was reliable, interested in them and willing to carry out even "unpleasant" tasks. A slow response . . . often became the starting point for diminished trust in the reliability of all care procedures; it kindled latent resentment; and it often constituted "proof" that the patient's demands were not taken seriously.[2]

[1]D. Tagliacozzo, "The Nurse from the Patients' Point of View," in Skipper, J., Jr., and Leonard R. (eds.), *Social Interaction and Patient Care*, Philadelphia, J. B. Lippincott Co., 1965, p. 224.

[2]Ibid., p. 225.

Briefly, nurses function on a caring-power continuum. The more they use caring tactics and the less they use power tactics, the more clients feel that their needs are met. The more clients' choices are considered, the less dependent and the less coerced by direct and subtle behaviors and attitudes they are made to feel.

Even though the study from which these quotations are taken was done in 1962, the conclusions, I believe, have serious, valid implications for today's practitioner. The client who feels dependent and powerless cannot be expected to "reveal his needs or . . . seize the initiative in obtaining the care which he desires or must have."[1] Clearly, in the hands of the nurse who uses power tactics, the client has little choice in sickness care.

Physicians' Selection

Perhaps the most obvious impediments to clients' exercising dying-related choices are their conscious and unconscious feelings about physicians. The natural desire to be well compels a person who becomes ill to seek a physician. Therefore, the potential client selects and visits a physician who the client hopes will facilitate a return to health. Clinical competence is paramount. Other very important considerations include the physician's manner of interacting with clients.

This selection is made in one of three ways. First, a friend or relative suggests a physician known by reputation or by a positive direct experience. Second, physicians frequently refer their clients to a colleague in another specialty. Third, by calling the local medical society, the potential client receives three random names in a particular field of medicine.

Only in the case of impending death will this individual have to consider whether the physician's and the nurses' beliefs will help or hinder his or her manner of dying. Has one chosen the physician whose philosophy regarding living and dying most closely resembles one's own? This information plus the educational and experiential background of the physician would enable the potential client to make a more informed decision. This information is usually not considered in selecting the physician.

In the future, with the increasing use of computers, it may be possible to record everyone's psychological profile. With participation by physicians and other providers of health care services, recipient and provider of care might be matched more advantageously. The frightening implications may be reduced by strict regulation. Several important considerations, such as privacy safeguards, a high degree of tool accuracy, and a mechanism for periodic updates, would be necessary.

Recently, the consumer health movement has proposed the publication of directories of physicians that would include academic and experiential background and professional and client evaluations of interpersonal and technical skills. There are flaws in this system also, but it is an improvement over the

[1]Ibid., p. 226.

traditional methods. One obvious flaw is in the evaluation. A physician might choose to include only favorable client and collegial evaluations.

For those people choosing not to be computerized or published in directories, the currently conventional methods of physician selection via referrals from friend, relative, physician, or local medical society would operate. Those clients not using the computer or directories would have a special need for an advocate.

Physicians' Aura

After choosing physicians by any one of the currently available methods, clients now have even less opportunity for choices. Many clients, both lay and professional, are hypnotized by the aura of the physician. Because the physician is perceived as the expert, blind faith is placed in that person's decisions.

Clients frequently ask very few questions of physicians, thereby accepting everything that is done to and for them as necessary. Some clients have such great faith in their physicians that no questions are necessary. They really believe that physicians will give them all the necessary information without their asking questions. These clients truly relinquish all choice in their treatment. Often, queries are not made because of the subservient, psychologically and physically submissive position in which clients are placed. When doctors appear too busy, clients do not interrupt. Conversation with clients often entails the use of medical terminology unfamiliar to them. Upon entering a client's room, physicians often remain at a physical distance from the client and thereby promote psychological distance. The result is physician-controlled communication. Often physicians converse directly with nearby professional staff to the exclusion of the clients who are also nearby. Ignored clients do not feel comfortable enough to interrupt "important" conversations. Anxiety and physician aura often cause clients to forget questions they wanted to ask.

Clients also try to assess their physicians' moods. If physicians are perceived as ill-tempered, clients ask no questions and thereby avoid threatening the physician-client relationship. This relationship, moreover, is strained by many other factors, as the following quotation will indicate:

> Patients often voice the following complaints about their physician: (1) high costs; (2) not enough genuine interest; too impersonal; (3) inadequate personal respect; (4) examinations too hurried; (5) insufficient discussion of findings, diagnosis, treatment, and prognosis; (6) excessive waiting in office; (7) too much delay in appointments (some complain of too many appointments); (8) inaccessibility during office hours; (9) too little interest, consideration, and aid from office assistants; (10) too little or too much consultation; (11) implication or designation of troubles as psychiatric; (12) too old or too young; (13) too unknowledgeable; and (14) "I just don't like him." Many of these problems are related to the physician's failure to orient the patient and key members of his family and win their friendship, respect and full cooperation. When the patient understands the significance and possible benefits of certain diagnostic and therapeutic procedures, he is less bothered by

the time, cost, and effort involved. He also tends to become more relaxed and cooperative, more loyal to and respectful of his physician.[1]

To overcome the communication-stifling physician aura, nurses can effectively act as client advocates. Simply by translating terminology unfamiliar to clients, they can reduce anxiety. Assistance should be given to forgetful clients by helping them to prepare a list of questions before the physicians' visit. Of course, reminding clients of the previously prepared lists of questions during the physician's visit may also be necessary.

House Service Clients

Individuals entering teaching hospitals expect to receive the most up-to-date care. Certainly, once admitted to the hospital, they usually do receive the most advanced, although possibly the least individualized, care. This situation occurs because these service institutions maintain close relationships with the educational and research communities. Clients' individual needs are often secondary to the need of interns and residents to learn. "This conflict in value system is greatest for the practitioner who cares for . . . his patients in a university hospital, devoted to the development, evaluation, and application of the most advanced medical technology."[2]

Very little difference in care exists between a person entering the hospital who has a private physician and a person who does not have a private physician. The private physician, if available, remains ultimately responsible but serves as consultant and sometimes as teacher to the interns and residents. For the person without a private physician, who is called a *house service* or *ward "patient,"* the consultant and teacher for the interns and residents is usually a highly qualified physician with many years of experience in medicine and a strong interest in teaching.

After the client is introduced to the house officer on duty, the client's choices now diminish further. The two choices remaining are either (1) if able, to leave the hospital against medical advice or (2) to accept the whole hospitalization package. This may also be true for non–house service clients. Many consent forms, except those forms for special procedures, give the physician carte blanche to do as he or she chooses. The intern or resident decides on the appropriate diagnostic and treatment modalities.

Because fledgling doctors need experience in new techniques, they may consciously or unconsciously omit giving clients facts necessary to make an informed decision about a possibly life-threatening treatment or diagnostic procedure, such as cardiac catheterization. Depending upon the sensitivity, interests, and feelings of the intern or resident and the direction provided by the

[1]R. Williams, "Sick with Kindness, Compassion, Wisdom and Efficiency," in Williams, R. (ed.), *To Live and to Die: When, Why, and How*, New York, Springer-Verlag, 1973, p. 143.
[2]D. and L. Rabin, "Consequences of Death for Physicians, Nurses and Hospitals," in Brim, O., Jr. (ed.), *The Dying Patient*, New York, Russell Sage Foundation, 1970, p. 181.

private physician, the client's interests and feelings may or may not be considered. In recent years the issue of informed consent has been looked at anew. How much information does the client need to give informed consent?

With the recent consumer movement, more clients are becoming aware of their rights to accept or refuse care, but violations still exist. Many students in the health care professions still learn their skills without asking clients' permission. Clients may experience, in addition, ambivalence toward students in that while they understand the need to learn, they do not want to be the person with whom the students practice. On the other hand, some clients prefer students because they will often spend more time with them than physicians will.

By the time the medical student has become an intern, dying has become impersonal. The corpse is a former diagnosis on whom attempts at treatment have failed—a medical curiosity to be dissected. "For the [first-year] student, the cadaver is primarily a machine with whose pieces and parts he must become thoroughly familiar if he is to pass his anatomy examinations."[1] To many physicians a death is a professional failure. Feifel feels that physicians have a stronger fear of death than their clients do. Given the difficulties physicians experience in caring for the dying client, the problem still remains, How can a person die peacefully in a hospital dedicated to cure and rehabilitation?

Whether or not the client is dying, one must consider that hospitals function on a cure-rehabilitation philosophy. Therefore, for its responsibilities to be fulfilled, clients must submit to many kinds of therapies in order to regain some degree of wellness, whether or not the client is perceived as dying. When finally considered incurable, the client has usually been subjected to an exhaustive series of diagnostics and treatments. Of course his or her consent is assumed.

The situation in the smaller community hospitals differs due to the decreased number of interacting personnel. Individuals entering community hospitals also relinquish choices pertinent to their care, but these choices are relinquished directly to the attending physician. Depending on the quality of rapport and the duration of interaction, opportunity for direct dialogue with private physicians can be greater in the community hospital.

The difference in communication patterns in small and large groups may explain the increased opportunity for dialogue in the community hospital. Small and large groups as well as hospitals use formal communication channels and mechanisms to help maintain order and accomplish the tasks at hand. Clients understand that certain questions can be answered only by the physician while nurses are able to answer other types of questions. As the size of the group increases, more formalized and less personalized channels of communication become necessary. Although the tendency to formalize structure for efficiency and business purposes does exist in both types of hospitals, there are proportionately a smaller number of persons with whom to interact in a smaller community hospital. Therefore, clients' chances of being heard there may be

[1]Ibid., p. 173.

greater than in a larger teaching hospital. The majority of clients who die in institutions, moreover, die in community hospitals. Often they want to be close to home, loved ones, and neighbors and to have no more extra lifesaving measures (like the ones used in larger teaching hospitals) taken. Nevertheless, a good dialogue between client and health care workers clearly depends on the personalities involved and the rapport achieved between the two people, whether the dialogue be in a community or university hospital.

Lack of Privacy

Problems still exist in maintaining clients' privacy. To the degree that personal privacy is relinquished, autonomy and individuality are also diminished. Regardless of the type of hospital, clients' bodies, histories, illnesses, and treatments are open to any interested personnel. Dying clients are no exception.

The fishbowl atmosphere of the hospital is most obvious to clients who are interrupted by personnel wanting to perform some task when they are using the bedpan or urinal. The variety of interruptions extends from the physician making rounds to the kitchen employee removing or delivering a meal tray. The tasks of the hospital personnel continue around the often undressed client, who has completely lost privacy, dignity, and autonomy.

Another kind of privacy frequently violated by the health care team is the privacy of shared confidences, especially about personal affairs. In the planning of nursing care, confidential information may sometimes need to be shared with other health care team members. However, confidential information may be indiscretely shared with someone who does not need to know it. If the confidence is broken, the client risks humilation, anxiety, and loss of trust in the health care worker.

On occasion a physician or nurse may ask clients' permission before students observe or care for them. In allowing themselves to be studied, clients serve valuable teaching and learning functions for students. Usually, however, permission is not requested and clients are subjected to seen and unseen observers. Students gather around clients' bedsides during procedures such as liver biopsies and spinal punctures. However, anesthetized clients are unaware of students who are observing and, sometimes, assisting during surgery.

In recent years, hospitals have become more cautious about using clients for specially designated research studies. Clients must sign approval forms. Research studies are rigidly controlled. On the other hand, most clients are unaware that, after removal, portions of their bodies, such as tissue samples and dead fetuses, may also be used for research, especially in teaching hospitals.

Clients exercise little control over their charts. They assume their charts are utilized only by those people essential to their care, who have a need to know. Ideally and ethically this is true. However, charts are usually kept at the nurses' station, and anyone having access to or business at the nurses' station may open and read the chart. Clients' only recourse is to insist that their charts be kept in their rooms. Then anyone wishing to see them would have to ask permission of the clients. In reality, clients infrequently see their own charts. Clients should be made aware that they can ask to read the chart. While new laws in some states permit access to charts, there are still some difficulties in carrying out this process.

Hospital Discharge

The discharge power resides with physicians and utilization review committees, not with clients. For most hospitals the advent of Medicare initiated these committees, whose purpose is to prevent prolonged and unnecessary hospitalizations. Shortening hospitalization time makes more beds available for more admissions, thereby increasing hospital revenue.

As the time for discharge approaches, the physician, sometimes in collaboration with the nursing staff, determines date, time, mode of transportation, and posthospitalization placement. The client may not be consulted, but just told the time of departure. Families are restricted to providing transportation and care in their own or convalescent homes. Furthermore, when clients are medically ready for discharge, conflict often occurs between the physician and the utilization review committee because teaching or posthospitalization placement needs may not have been met.

The only way clients can be assured of leaving the hospital when they wish is by signing a disclaimer of liability for the hospital. By "signing out against medical advice" clients release the hospital from any responsibility for their well-being after discharge. This is not a routine matter. It requires a strong will and perseverance for clients to obtain this form from the hospital staff. Such an attempt implies a conflict of goals between physician and client.

By not making a decision to leave the hospital, clients can choose to die there by default. Once admitted to the hospital, though, those clients wishing to die at home may require special discharge arrangements. Clients can either sign a disclaimer of liability and leave the hospital or request the physician to officially discharge them. Plans must be made then for posthospitalization care either by the family alone or with assistance from health care personnel visiting the home.

Family's Role

Upon entering a hospital, families, like clients, feel they are trespassing on foreign territory. The sights, sounds, and smells of the hospital often frighten them.

Families are almost as dependent as clients upon the health care team of the hospital. They need information about rules and regulations, specifically about visiting hours. The only real difference in dependency between clients and families is mobility: Families can walk out freely at the end of visiting hours.

The only tangible way families can be reassured of the quality of care being given is to see if all the tasks are done properly. For instance, is the bedpan given without delay? Is the bed clean? Are the proper pills given on time? In addition to observing the tasks, families listen and remember every word the doctor or nurse says about prognosis, treatment, and progress. However, if the anxiety level of the families is too high, either they do not hear what is being said or they distort the message given. In times of uncertainty and stress, they cling to these words and tasks to maintain their equilibrium.

Traditionally, with the focus being almost exclusively on the client, the family's role has been limited to a short visit each day. Clients and families usually cannot choose the hours most suitable for visiting. Visiting hours are established by hospital policy, and this policy often forbids children under the age of 12 or 14 years to visit. Intensive care units limit visiting times to 5 or 10 minutes every hour. These hours are established around the work schedule of doctors and nurses. If visiting hours were to be allowed in the morning, visitors might interrupt physician "rounds" or a bed bath or treatment. Recently, some hospitals have become more flexible in their policies regarding visitors.

Actually, the family and a few personal possessions the clients keep in their rooms serve as the only links with the familiar outside world. Families can be invaluable in the care of clients. For clients unable to speak for themselves, families can provide information about clients' likes, dislikes, habits, and life-style. Families can also help orient clients. By sharing in the development of the health care plan, families are made to feel an important part of the hospitalization process. Families can be taught to perform treatments for clients if they desire, especially in preparation for posthospitalization care. There is nothing wrong in allowing family members to give a bed bath to clients if they desire. A trusting family is a powerful ally in client-centered care. Families can actually help keep clients' anxiety at a productive level.

During a prolonged or even a short illness families endure great stress. Nurses should be aware that they can alleviate family stress by suggesting that the family needs time away from the client to regain their strengths. An evening at a movie or a restaurant can provide the change needed to allow families to survive illnesses.

Sick Model

All human service professions function by assisting someone in need. Since someone is in need, there is a problem to be solved. The problem to the health care worker is illness.

Health care professions is a euphemism. They should more accurately be called *sickness care professions*. They function on a sick model, that is, focus on illness and detection of problems while minimizing the role of the well parts of the body. For example, the problem-oriented medical record was developed to more accurately identify the symptoms of illness, to record and chart the progress of treatment, and to list resolved problems. In the sick model, the existing problems are meant to be solved by the sickness care worker, who

plans and executes treatment. Clients' only choices are refusal
acceptance of care.

Even people entering the ambulatory care setting are immed
to as *patients*, that is, sick until proven well. Sickness care v
imagine clients seeking health maintenance services. For nurses, annual physical examinations are preliminary to diagnosis and treatment. Perhaps the ex-
pansion of health maintenance organizations that focus on health maintenance
and not just on detecting problems and the increased stress on disease prevention will tip the scale in favor of a more balanced and accurate approach
to clients.

The sick model frequently may see dying clients maladapting to the crisis
of dying. This maladaptation requires psychosocial intervention; for example,
if a dying client is observed to cry frequently and display anger at the nurses,
he or she is perceived as having a "problem." The nurse may ask for a consultation for the client with a psychiatrist to help solve the problem. Actually
it is the nurse and not the client who has the problem. Crying and anger are
very appropriate when a person is grieving about anticipated death.

Along with changes in terminology must go changes in attitudes. The
passive patient must become the active client working with the health care
team in meeting his or her needs. The client's rights must be respected. To
help change attitudes a client advocate may be necessary. Health care professionals in addition must increasingly look for the client's strengths and support
them, especially during illness. This is the key concept in the well model, which
will be discussed in the next chapter.

SUMMARY

Obstacles to the dying client's having choices in care pervade the sickness care
milieu. Care is formularized by the use of the "patient care plan," which
frequently presents the textbook picture of the client. Care plans need to be
more client-centered, reflecting the identity of the individual and how the disease
has affected this person. They must always be in process.

Psychological mechanisms, when misunderstood as all-or-nothing pre-
cepts, limit understanding of the very complex process of dying. The literature
is replete with examples of denial or acceptance of death as pervasive American
societal attitudes. Using denial or acceptance as unifying concepts or independent mental mechanisms around which dying should be viewed inhibits further
inquiry into other relevant characteristics of how our contemporary culture
views dying. It is like saying that an automobile runs on gasoline; it does, but
there are many other components needed for proper functioning of an
automobile.

Modern hospital and medical practice has presented many more obstacles
to a peaceful death. The most obvious obstacle is the hospital's primary goal
of cure and rehabilitation. Often the presence or behavior of the dying client

makes the nurse or other health care workers uncomfortable. Many avoidance patterns of nurses and other health care workers, such as moving the dying client to the end of the corridor, have been documented by Glaser and Strauss.

The aura of the hospital administration and bureaucratic constraints combine to reduce the sense of personal care and choice at the expense of efficiency. Clients and families are affected by the hospital administration's aura through hospital rules and regulations, such as visiting hours; through cursory visits by administrator to client; and through visits by the administrator due to medicolegal problems.

Nurses' perceptions of the dying person are developed by the educational institution's focus on cure, rehabilitation, and return to maximum functioning. The need for effective listening to the dying person is blocked by preconceived notions, stereotyped attitudes, and distorted perceptions.

Clients view nurses with sterotypical notions ranging from the image of the cold, efficient nurse to that of the angel of mercy in white. Being almost completely dependent upon the nurse, clients seek to be acceptable and pleasing and thereby to receive the needed care.

None of the typical ways a physician is selected considers the compatibility of the doctor and the client regarding issues of life and death. Most commonly physicians are chosen at the suggestion of a friend or relative, through collegial referral by the primary physician, or through referral by the local medical society of three random names. In the future, computers and published directories may assist in achieving a more compatible personality matching of health care workers and clients.

Physicians' aura may also be an obstacle to clients' choices about dying. Often, because physicians are perceived as an expert, blind faith is put in their decisions and few questions are asked by clients. Using distancing behavior, such as speaking in medical terminology, not approaching the client's bedside, and talking to professional staff instead of the client, increases the client's anxiety and stifles communication. If the client perceives the physician as ill-tempered or very busy, the client will also avoid communication.

The rules and responsibilities under which the house staff personnel must function diminish choice, control, and dignity of clients in their illness-related care. The educational and research needs of interns and residents can take precedence over personalized client care. Many consent forms give carte blanche to do as the physicians choose. Some clients are aware of the right to refuse care since the advent of the consumer movement.

House service clients, in particular in large teaching hospitals, are given less choice in their care than are clients who receive care by a private physician in a smaller community hospital. Smaller community hospitals, in contrast to large teaching institutions, may be more willing to give personalized care because of their proportionately less bureaucratization and personnel.

Even with the consumer movement there are still problems in maintaining the client's privacy. Bodily, legal, treatment, and interpersonal privacy may be violated as the client is used as an object for learning, teaching, or just sharing information indiscriminately.

Discharge-making decisions are customarily at the discretion of the attending physician and the utilization review committee. If the client wishes to go home and the physician does not agree, the client's only recourse is to "sign out against medical advice" and release the hospital of any legal responsibility.

Families, like clients, also are dependent upon the health care worker. They need information about and care for their hospitalized relative. Experiencing great stress when a family member is hospitalized, families need more consideration from personnel than they now receive. A close family can be a useful adjunct to nursing care in keeping the client calm, reassured, and cooperative.

The most pervasive and least obvious obstacle to client-centered care of the dying is the focus of the entire team on the sick model, that is, on looking for problems, treating them, and discarding the well aspects of the person.

Along with changing terminology must go changing attitudes. Clients' rights must be more scrupulously safeguarded. An advocate may be needed. In addition to the client's problems, we must identify the client's innate and acquired strengths and support them, especially in the case of the dying client.

QUESTIONS FOR REFLECTION AND DISCUSSION

2-1 If you could pick the manner in which you preferred to die, what would be your choice?

2-2 What would you do if you could write your own death certificate?

2-3 How would you write your own obiturary and eulogy?

2-4 List the news stories relating to death and dying for the past week. In what manner were they presented by the media?

2-5 Read or view some fictional accounts of dying. In what manner were they presented by the media?

2-6 Have you ever attended a wake or a funeral? If so, what were your reactions to the deceased and to the people around you? What were the other mourners' reactions?

2-7 What are some of the rites and rituals in your family surrounding death?

2-8 Ask five of your colleagues, both students and graduate nurses, what they would do and say to "reassure" or "provide emotional support" for a client who is going to surgery for a breast biopsy. What would you say? What would be the best thing to say? (This question provides an opportunity for role playing.)

2-9 Ask three physicians if and how they tell their clients a terminal diagnosis. What contingencies make revealing a diagnosis most difficult? What is the physician's most vivid experience with death? Why? What does the physician think the nurse's role is and the most difficult aspects of that role are in caring for a dying client? Choose physicians with varying backgrounds.

2-10 Ask five clients how they chose their doctors. Is there a better way? Ask these clients how they feel about their doctors.

2-11 Ask your hospital administrator how clients' rights are protected. Is this adequate?
2-12 What is the policy in your hospital about the client seeing the chart? Can the client keep it in his or her room?
2-13 Identify five ways you could be a better client advocate. Give examples.
2-14 Identify five ways a client can be given more choice in care.
2-15 Does your hospital have a patient representative? What are this person's duties? How effective is he or she? Is the representative paid by the hospital? If so, might there be a conflict of interest? How can this conflict of interest be avoided?

BIBLIOGRAPHY

Becker, E.: *The Denial of Death*, New York, Free Press, 1973.

Bloch, D.: "Privacy," in Carlson, C. E. (ed.), *Behavioral Concepts and Nursing Intervention*, Philadelphia, J. B. Lippincott Co., 1970.

Dumont, R., and Foss, D.: *The American View of Death: Acceptance or Denial*, Cambridge, Mass., Schenkman Publishing Co., 1972.

Feifel, H.: "Death," in Farberow, N. (ed.), *Taboo Topics*, New York, Atherton Press, 1963.

——— (ed.): *The Meaning of Death*, New York, McGraw-Hill Book Co., 1959.

Hinton, J.: *Dying*, Baltimore, Pelican Press, 1967.

"How to Develop a Local Directory of Doctors," *Consumer Reports*, **39**(9):685–691, September 1974.

"How to Find a Doctor for Yourself," *Consumer Reports*, **39**(9):681–684, September 1974.

Janken, J.: "The Nurse in Crisis," *The Nursing Clinics of North America*, **9**(1):17–26, March 1974.

Kübler-Ross, E.: *On Death and Dying*, New York, Macmillan Co., 1969.

Levinson, R.: "Sexism in Medicine," *American Journal of Nursing*, **76**(3):426–431, March 1976.

Mannes, M.: *Last Rites, A Case for the Good Death*, New York, William Morrow and Co., 1974.

Mauksch, H.: "The Nurse: Coordinator of Patient Care," in Skipper, J., Jr., and Leonard, R. (eds.), *Social Interaction and Patient Care*, Philadelphia, J. B. Lippincott Co., 1965.

Phillips, D.: "The Hospital and the Dying Patient," *Hospitals, Journal of American Hospital Association*, **46**:68–75, February 1972.

Quinn, N., and Somers, A.: "The Patient's Bill of Rights, A Significant Aspect of the Consumer Revolution," *Nursing Outlook*, **22**(2):240–444, April 1974.

Rabin, D. and L.: "Consequences of Death for Physicians, Nurses and Hospitals," in Brim, O., Jr., et al. (eds.), *The Dying Patient*, New York, Russell Sage Foundation, 1970.

Smith, D.: "Patienthood and Its Threat to Privacy," *American Journal of Nursing*, **69**(3):509–513, March 1969.

Sudnow, D.: *Passing On*, Englewood Cliffs, N.J., Prentice-Hall, 1967.

Tagliacozzo, D.: "The Nurse from the Patient's Point of View," in Skipper, J., Jr., and Leonard, R. (eds.), *Social Interaction and Patient Care*, Philadelphia, J. B. Lippincott Co., 1965.

Weisman, A.: *On Dying and Denying*, New York, Behavioral Publications, 1972.
————: *The Realization of Death*, New York, Jason Aronson, 1974.
Williams, R.: "Sick with Kindness, Compassion, Wisdom and Efficiency," in Williams,
    R. (ed.), *To Live and to die: When, Why and How*, New York, Springer-Verlag,
    1973.
Zind, R.: "Deterrants to Crisis Intervention in the Hospital Unit," *The Nursing Clinics
    of North America*, **9**(1):27–36, March 1974.

Chapter 3

The Well Model

As mentioned in the previous chapter, health care workers have functioned on the sick model. They have had patients who were assumed to be "sick" because they sought help for physical problems. The patient was a passive recipient of care. The sick model compartmentalizes, pigeonholes, and seeks to cure because it can see only the effects of illness. However, illness is only one part of the lifecycle. Nursing need no longer function on the sick, or medical, model. For that matter, medicine need no longer function on the sick model.

One takes on the sick role after one views oneself as having an illness. Sociologically, Parsons discusses the institutionalized view of the sick role. First, it is a right and an obligation of a sick person to be exempted from normal social role responsibilities. Second, a sick person cannot get better alone and must seek help. Third, being ill is undesirable, and the person is obliged to get well. Fourth, he or she must seek competent help and must cooperate in his or her care.

However, it is now necessary to consider patients as clients, being represented by a professional person, being active participants, and making significant choices in their care, if health care professions are to meet clients' real needs. The strengths all clients possess, even at a time of great crisis, can and should be used for support when their sense of equilibrium and stability is shaken. For some dying clients, for instance, religion becomes a strong support, bringing a measure of peace.

In explaining the well model, we will first define the essential terms and concepts used throughout the chapter and the book, including the special problem of maladaptation. The second part of the chapter is devoted to the axioms or assumptions upon which the well model is based. These axioms are not meant to include a comprehensive discussion of the ideas of every positivist philosopher, social scientist, or biologist, but to be examples of the large number of similar views of human beings as potentially self-actualizing. This is not to deny that humans have destructive potential, for certainly human beings fulfill themselves through both productive and destructive expressions every day. The third part of the chapter applies the well model, schematically adapted to Lewin's field theory, to describe client interactions. Brief quotations are presented only to illustrate a point and to more clearly explain an axiom.

ESSENTIAL TERMS AND CONCEPTS

In developing the well model, I investigated the areas of physiological and psychological stress and crisis theory. These fields are fraught with semantic problems. What is considered to be stress in one model is not stress in another. The similarities are as confusing as the differences. (The reader with a special interest in these areas will find the readings at the end of the chapter helpful.) With these semantic problems in mind, and for the purpose of this book, the terms *health* and *wellness, adaptation, stress, equilibrium, margin of equilibrium safety*, and *sickness* will be defined.

Health to most people is expressed in terms of ability to perform life tasks. Health and its synonym, *wellness*, are abstract concepts seen only in their physical, psychological, and social manifestations. As an absolute, health does not exist. Since any definition is limited by the criteria used to measure the concept and since the criteria for measuring health are vague, the definition of health will remain vague until more precise measurements are established.

For the purpose of this book *health is defined as a process and a function of the person's innate and learned capacities to maintain maximum well-being in all systems and spheres of existence including the essential interplay of internal and external environments*. It is possible to be healthy and, therefore, to function if a person has diabetes, a colostomy, or paraplegia. The definition of health for each person rests upon the personal perception of the tasks necessary for adequate living.

Adaptation is a unifying mechanism by which a person flexibly integrates new experiences consciously and unconsciously.

Because of the semantic problems in stress research, *stress is used to mean any effect on the body initiating an adaptive change*. Stress can be called *strain, vector, need, anxiety, force*, or *illness*. Stress can be pleasant or unpleasant.

In effect, equilibrium and adaptation are processes through which a degree of health is maintained. *Equilibrium in the living organism is a dynamic, moving,*

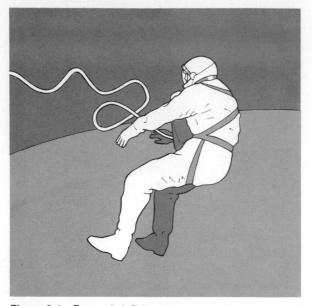

Figure 3-1   Person in infinite environment with support systems.

never absolute process of varying degrees in which the organism shifts its internal and external environments for the purpose of maintaining integrity and life processes. Health is also a concept in which seemingly contradictory words, *stability* and *change*, are blended. Moreover, equilibrium is both a goal and a process related to developmental and situational circumstances. Since "process is a dynamic term denoting change,"[1] maintenance of equilibrium cannot be considered as maintenance of the status quo, but must be considered in terms of growth, becoming, creativity, and potential. "In the process of becoming, potentialities are actualized. Actualization does not fulfill the totality of potentialities present. There is uncertainty in the nature of the change that may occur. Change is unidirectional and not predetermined."[2] In other words, although a person is always becoming and future-oriented, the changes are not preset by any force and are not predictable.

There is a margin of equilibrium safety that can be considered healthy, that is, not leading to disorganization and collapse. Consider the space-walking astronauts (Figure 3-1), who had a finite margin of equilibrium safety—the end of the rope—in an infinite environment. Beyond that rope were disintegration and death. Life-support systems, including the rope, helped maintain equilibrium while the person was under the stress of an unfamiliar and hostile envi-

---

[1]M. Rogers, *An Introduction to the Theoretical Basis of Nursing*, Philadelphia, F. A. Davis Co., 1970, p. 9.
    [2]Ibid., p. 58.

ronment. We all have finite margins of equilibrium safety, or end points beyond which we collapse and disintegrate. The margin of equilibrium safety, the rope's end, may be different for each person (Figure 3-2). *The margin of equilibrium safety, therefore, can be defined as the point of equilibrium beyond which disintegration, collapse, and subsequently death occur.*

Sickness can be defined only in terms of distance from the margin of equilibrium safety. *Therefore, sickness is defined as a process and a function of the disequilibrium reaction to circumstances in the internal and external environments that may lead to disorganization and collapse.* A circumstance can be called a *force, vector, need, discomfort, tension, strain, stress,* or *crisis* depending upon the degree of intensity of the stimulus.

Circumstances act as stressors, initiating coping mechanisms. Sickness does not always lead to collapse, but can be a growth-producing process by which inner and outer resources are utilized to improve even a previously high level of well-being. The person, for example, with appendicitis does not necessarily collapse and die. The internal biological resources are mobilized to defend the body against infection. The external resources employed may be members of the health care professions, family, and other significant supports.

Another example of illness producing growth can be seen in the recovery of the mastectomy client. Psychodynamically the illness produces grief whose resolution evolves through intra-psychic processes and social supports. As the client recovers she finds she has gained strength and personal growth from the experience. In other words, she has integrated the experience and become an even more fully functional human being.

Figure 3-2   Boundary of acceptable living.

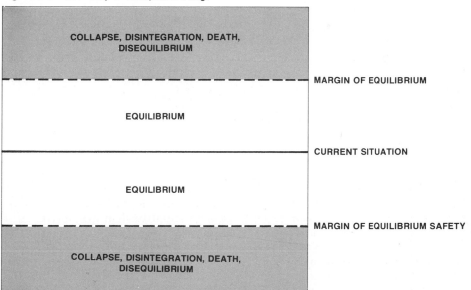

THE PROBLEM OF MALADAPTATION

In a review of the literature on physiological, psychological, and social aspects of stress, grief, and crisis theory, the term *maladaptation* is used to describe an inability to cope adequately with stress, leading to disequilibrium and disorganization. It is definitely not a growth-producing phenomenon, but it is often not clear whether *maladaptation* refers to the process of reacting, is the result of the reaction, or both.

On this term hangs an onerous value judgment. Maladaptive behavior, compared with acceptable and therefore good behavior, is found to be deficient. The word *maladaptive* implicitly blames the victim.

Frequently, the person in extreme distress finds his usual coping patterns inadequate to the present task. There is then an inverse relationship between the potency of the stress and the ability of the body to defend against it. An increased anxiety level starts a cycle of less and less adequate coping responses. This is not maladaptive behavior but is a weakening of current ability to function brought on by the degree of stress. As the degree of stress and tension increases, the person sees fewer and fewer choices available for action. At the height of the stress he or she sees no more choices. Disorganization, not maladaptation, occurs. The person is adapting in the only way available. The term *maladaptation* should not be used. The body *may* react in direct proportion to the potency of the stress; then a balanced state exists. While *coping* implies successful overcoming of a challenge through a struggle, it is not a synonym for *adapting*, but adapting and coping are complementary in that the same end can be achieved through different means. Adaptation demands flexibility. The person who cannot cope well enough to maintain equilibrium is adapting unsuccessfully. Maladaptation does not exist.

BASIC ASSUMPTIONS OF THE WELL MODEL

The well model is presented as a more positive way of thinking about client care. Underlying the concepts of the well model are certain assumptions about the relationship of human beings to each other, but most especially, the assumptions identify the need of individuals to fulfill themselves. By nature human beings are innovative.

1 Human beings have a special uniqueness seen only when one observes their totality.

The usual way of analyzing human beings, in the sick model, is in terms of systems or compartments—the physical, psychological, social, spiritual, cultural, and many other levels. This cookbook approach allows only a partial view of human beings and their abilities; in other words, segmenting of tasks obscures the relationship of parts to the whole. The impact of a situation often cannot be seen in the breakdown of its component parts. The separate systems of the body, for instance, have little value unless their essential relationships can be viewed in the context of the entire body. By looking at the total person one recognizes that all parts appear important, and their essential relationships are discernible.

This assumption is basic to both the well model and nursing. "Man is a unified whole possessing his own integrity and manifesting characteristics that are more than and different from the sum of his parts."[1] It is much easier to understand wholeness, in contrast with segmentation in discussing human emotions. Love and hate cannot be compartmentalized because they are total responses of a person. Human integrity and dignity also do not exist separated into parts.

On a more pathological or disequilibrium level, many concepts can be understood only in their totality because the response of the person is total; for example, when specific nerve endings are damaged, the person in pain responds with the whole self. The mind is centered on the pain, and body functions are totally directed toward relieving it. The person in respiratory distress, likewise, can think of nothing else but breathing. His or her reaction is total.

In terms of rapid sociological change, Toffler refers to *future shock* as a total phenomenon defined as "distress, both physical and psychological, that arises from an overload of the human organism's physical adaptive system, and its decision-making process . . . the human response to overstimulation."[2] In discussing new graduate nurses' reactions to the work environment, Kramer defines *reality shock* as the "total social, physical, and emotional response of a person to the unexpected, unwanted, or undesired, and in the most severe degree to the intolerable."[3]

From the physiological perspective, Selye now defines *stress* as "the non-specific response of the body to any demand made upon it" in contrast with his earlier definition, "the *sum* of all non-specific changes caused by function or damage."[4] He implies that stree has a quality that is different from the individual changes in the body.

2   The well model assumes that the natural tendency of each person is toward at least survival and at most health and equilibrium:

> As long as a person maintains the integrity and uniqueness of his individual nature, growth of the self (which begins at birth) continues throughout life. The urge to express one's individual nature and come to full self-realization lies within each person. It is neither a quiescent drive that must be activated by external pressures and motivations nor an effort to relieve tensions. On the contrary, the urge to become is a positive force. . . . The self by its nature is inclined to grow and move toward an evolving identity and an individuality that has an irrevocable biological basis.[5]

In contrast, the sick model views the person as ill, and survival depends upon intervention of health care persons. We must give more emphasis to the

[1]Ibid., p. 47.
[2]A. Toffler, *Future Shock*, New York, Random House, 1970, p. 326.
[3]M. Kramer, *Reality Shock*, St. Louis, C. V. Mosby Co., 1974, pp. 3–4.
[4]H. Selye, *Stress without Distress*, Philadelphia, J. B. Lippincott Co., 1974, p. 141.
[5]C. Moustakas, *Creativity and Conformity*, New York, D. Van Nostrand Co., 1967, p. 2.

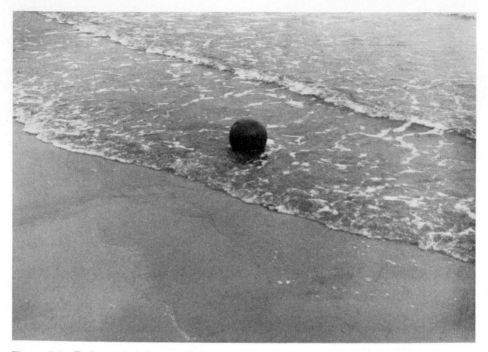

Figure 3-3 To be carried along by life's current is to drift toward fulfillment and peace.

individual's personal resources. Life is a changing and unidirectional process. Through the exercise of free will, one can reverse the drive toward survival and bring destruction upon oneself. Technological advances cannot assure human beings of survival and, in fact, can destroy us. In a few years our water may be undrinkable; some people believe it is now. The number of automobile accidents is proof that our technological advances do not always function to our advantage. You may be able to get to a destination faster, but the automobile also enables you to kill yourself faster. "While choice can be made more rational by basing it on factual information, on evaluation of consequences, it always retains a personal component because it must ultimately involve a value judgment."[1] Motivation to choose between growth-producing behavior and destructive behavior is determined, according to Maslow, by our basic needs. If our basic needs are fulfilled we feel safe to grow to yet another level of development. When these basic needs—now called *deficiency needs*, are left unmet, these "empty holes . . . must be filled up for health's sake . . . from without by human beings other than the subject."[2]

Healthy people have sufficiently gratified their basic needs for safety, belongingness, love, respect and self-esteem so that they are motivated primarily by trends of self-actualization (defined as ongoing actualization of potentials, capacities and

[1]R. Dubos, *So Human an Animal*, New York, Charles Scribner's Sons, 1968, p. 131.
[2]A. Maslow, *Toward a Psychology of Being*, New York, D. Van Nostrand Reinhold Co., 1968, pp. 22–23.

talents as fulfillment of mission or call, fate, destiny, or vocation), as a fuller knowledge of, and acceptance of, the person's own intrinsic nature, as an unceasing trend toward unity, integration or synergy within the person.[1]

The belief in the value of and the innate drive for survival must be the basis of the therapeutic process and relationship. For without this belief, therapy would be purposeless. Carl Rogers' view of himself as a therapeutic agent is well stated: ''If I can provide a certain type of relationship, the other person will discover within himself the capacity to use that relationship for growth, and change and personal development will occur.''[2] Since our beginnings, human beings have constantly striven to fulfill their potentials. Bronowski cites many examples of our use of our imaginative gifts to progressively enrich ourselves and the world in areas such as art, music, and science.

3   Wellness or health and, therefore, survival, are dependent upon the ability of the person to adapt.

Adaptation as a unifying phenomenon is essential for survival. More specifically, it is the mechanism by which life processes are integrated so that health and growth are maintained.

Evolution as a historical form of adaptation was first postulated by Darwin to meet, both biologically and socially, more or less permanent but changing needs:

> But man can and does select the variations given to him by nature, and thus accumulates them in any desired manner. He thus adapts animals and plants for his own benefit or pleasure. He may do this methodically or he may do it unconsciously by preserving the individuals most useful or pleasing to him.[3]

Whether in the development of jaw structure or of family structure, adaptation and refinement are the tools of evolution:

> The ability to change is a fundamental characteristic of life. But to be compatible with the continuance of life, any change must become harmoniously integrated with the various structures and functions that the organism has inherited from its evolutionary past. Life is historical, and it can continue only if the new becomes part of the old, or, at least, does not conflict too violently with the established order. One of the characteristics of life is that the past survives in the present and determines the acceptability of any change, just as the future determines its viability.[4]

The physiological adaptation capacity has been documented by Selye, who called it the *general adaptation syndrome* or the *biological stress syndrome*. It has three stages. The first stage is alarm, in which there is perception of the event and immediate efforts to neutralize the stressor. When these efforts are ineffective the second stage, resistance, occurs, in which a more or less total

[1]Ibid., p. 25.
[2]C. Rogers, *On Becoming a Person*, Boston, Houghton Mifflin Co., 1961, p. 13.
[3]C. Darwin, *The Origin of Species*, New York, Everyman's Library, 1928, p. 444.
[4]R. Dubos, *The Torch of Life*, New York, Simon & Schuster, 1962, p. 36.

effort is expended to bring the organism into .equilibrium or balance. If the second stage is inadequate the third stage, exhaustion and death, occurs. Obviously, exhaustion is disequilibrium.

I believe this third stage is not maladaptation, as Selye calls it, and as the sick model views it but under the circumstances is the only path left to the organism and therefore is adaptation. Exhaustion occurs due to either the inadequacy of the resistance factors or to the noxiousness of the stressor. An organism can tolerate these extreme conditions for only a short time.

The general adaptation syndrome is loosely analogous, although not usually identifiable as such, to crisis intervention theory in psychology. The first stage of crisis, Selye's alarm stage, includes perception of the hazardous event, an increase of tension, and mobilization of customary problem-solving measures. If these efforts are unsuccessful, the second or resistance stage, in which an all-out effort is made to thwart the stressor, is activated when emergency problem-solving measures are used. If these measures do not bring a resolution, redefinition of the problem is necessary to make it easier to solve or actual relinquishment of goals may be needed to reduce the stress. Finally, if none of the above measures helps, the third stage—maladaptation, collapse, and death—leads analogously to the crisis model's disorganization and collapse.

If the first two stages of the crisis model's attempt to restore the psychological equilibrium are unsuccessful, disorganization results. An unresolved crisis can be a prelude to suicide or homicide because potential options for action are so completely reduced. Both crisis-intervention theory and Selye's general adaptation syndrome are explicitly time-limited, but at any point before disorganization the client has an increased receptivity to intervention. No one has infinite ability to cope with seemingly endless or at least prolonged extreme stress. Disorganization and its consequences are inevitable.

4   Basic to the well model is the belief that each person is responsible for his or her own actions.

Legally, unless mentally incompetent, each person is expected to answer for his own actions. The United States Constitution and democracy are based upon the premise that each individual is important and is guaranteed the right to life, liberty, and the pursuit of happiness. This premise implies reponsibility and choice for without responsibility freedom becomes chaos.

Physicians and nurses functioning within the sick model have emasculated this inherent freedom and have chosen to take total responsibility for the client's care. The client's role is to follow orders and a treatment plan.

The Patient's Bill of Rights (reprinted in Appendix A) is based precisely on this assumption of responsibility. It is the responsibility of medicine and nursing to implement this document. To return autonomy to the client, the concept of self-responsibility must be internalized by every member of the medical and nursing professions. When this happens the client is free to be responsible. "The ability to choose among ideas and possible courses of action may be the most important to all human attributes; it has probably been and still is the crucial determinant of human evolution."[1]

5   Learning increases a person's strengths or potentials. Everyone is born with a specific genetic endowment. Nurture and its counterpart, education,

[1]Dubos, *So Human an Animal*, op. cit., p. 128.

develop this endowment. If this assumption were not generally accepted and prized, the entire system of formal education and the role of parents would be meaningless.

From the earliest times, parents have taught their children the rudiments of survival, such as how to obtain shelter and food. Much later, educational theory, from Plato and Socrates through the centuries to Comenius, Locke, Rousseau, Pestalozzi, Dewey, and Montessori, taught the value of education as a way to improve a person's ability to survive.

For nurses, this assumption is essential to client care. Without teaching and learning, few diabetics would survive long after their initial diagnosis. Diabetics would be forced to adapt without any new knowledge to help them cope with their disease. Learning has occurred when behavior has changed as a result of a newly integrated experience.

Preoperative teaching of the client can be thought of as anticipatory guidance with the goal of reducing future threat. By thinking through an impending situation, the client can initiate problem solving and can plan new healthy ways of coping.

In practice, preoperative teaching can reduce postoperative anxiety and the need for analgesics. Postoperative complications are reduced because clients perform necessary exercises without needing so much encouragement. Generally, preoperative teaching, both individual and group, significantly improves clients' speed of recovery from surgery. Client and family teaching is also helpful in other areas of nursing practice, for instance, obstetrics. Finally, by increasing a client's strengths through education, the nurse gives control back to the client, who should have had it in the first place.

6   Stress is normal and necessary for growth and development.

"Stress is the common denominator of all adaptive reactions of the body."[1] It is a necessary factor in survival. The complete absence of stress is stagnation and death. Even during sleep the body functions under a degree of stress to maintain life functions.

Stress, genetic endowment, and nurture are the essential ingredients for human fulfillment. Not only is a physically healthy body necessary for survival but an ability to adapt that body to changing circumstances is also essential. Psychologically, an attitude of eagerness to meet and adapt to change and challenge is also imperative.

In other words, people look for a challenge. Not only are people goal-oriented but also they constantly seek to become self-actualized, that is, to utilize potentials to the fullest. One's drive to fulfill oneself is innate. Constantly meeting and overcoming challenges, according to Maslow, begins with physical well-being and progresses to safety, social satisfaction, esteem, and finally self-actualization.

7   The well model assumes that individuals adapt to specific stressors in different ways. "We see indefinite variability in the endless slight peculiarities which distinguish the individuals of the same species, and which cannot be accounted for by inheritance from either parent or from some remote ancestor."[2] Given the endless variability of individuals, one can assume that there

[1]H. Selye, *The Stress of Life*, New York, McGraw-Hill Book Co., 1956, p. 54.
[2]Darwin, op. cit., p. 22.

is an endless variability in the ability to withstand stress. This difference in turn led Darwin to postulate the concept of survival of the fittest. A more recent example of variability of reactions to stress and the survival of the fittest is described in Piers Paul Read's *Alive*, the true story of an airplane crash of rugby players in the Chilean Andes mountains. The emotionally and physically weaker perished, while the stronger members fought to survive under seemingly impossible conditions.

There are many variables determining an individual's reaction to stress. The maturational level in large part determines the perceived intensity of threat in a given situation. To a 1-year-old child, a long stairway is a major threat to mobility. To an adult a stairway is just a means to get from one level to another.

Many kinds of coping behaviors can be mobilized to thwart the effects of stress on a person. A simple coping response to cold weather is to put on extra layers of clothing. Another coping response is that, physiologically, the perception of cold on the skin causes vasoconstriction to help retain body heat.

Environmental supports help a person adapt to stress. A familiar environment helps the geriatric client maintain a sense of integrity and orientation. Elderly clients quickly become confused when moved to different hospitals or even different rooms.

Maturational or developmental level in relation to reaction to stress can be considered from a physiological, psychological, and social viewpoint. The stress of rapid maturation, during early childhood and adolescence, for example, may diminish the ability of the person to cope with other stresses, such as physical ones. When a small child is mastering walking, speech development may temporarily slacken or moderate. Selye finds that in the second state of resistance

> resistance to a particular agent (in walking it is neuromuscular control) . . . is at its peak. . . . At the same time, resistance to most other agents (for instance, speech mastery) tends to fall below normal. It seems that the adjustment of our tissues to perform one function (detracts) from their adaptability to new circumstances.[1]

With the decreased intensity of stress (increased walking ability), the body is able to meet some other stressor (talking) in the body.

Psychological maturation can be described by considering the increasing gratification and self-confidence of the child who completes a series of tasks, for example, yearly promotion in school. The child who cannot complete these tasks as classmates do lacks gratification and self-confidence. The child who stays in the same grade for several years may not be able to focus on anything except his or her intellectual inability. Lack of success brings more lack of success. According to crisis theory, an increase in anxiety brought on by repeated years in the same grade makes the perceptual field become limited, and attempts at resolution of the problem become more remote without help. The person who meets with success in school gains confidence, and this confidence is a factor in success in dealing with other stresses.

Socially, the shifting of dependent, interdependent, and independent roles in relationships with other people can be viewed developmentally. The infant

---

[1]Selye, *The Stress of Life*, op. cit., p. 227.

is completely dependent on the parent. As the child grows, more indep
is achieved. The person who has not experienced warm, dependent relati
as a child may not be able to give in a warm relationship as an adult. The
needs to understand that he or she functions independently as a decision m..ker,
dependently as a consumer of essential products, and interdependently as a
family member:

> The concepts of maturity and adaptability are interlinked with concepts of potential
> for effective social functioning in much the same way that the concepts of growth
> and development are related to human potential for physical, mental, and emotional
> well-being.[1]

There are many factors influencing a person's ability to withstand stress.
What to one person is a problem of crisis proportions may be an easily resolved
situation to another.

For nurses, the variability of stress reactions makes client sickness care
more demanding and potentially more rewarding. It is part of the nursing process
to (1) identify the stress and its intensity, (2) discover how the client copes,
and (3) implement a plan of care to assist the client during the stressful event.

THE WELL MODEL

The well model assumes that people adapt to a particular set of circumstances
with a set of physiological, psychological, and situational potentials. One does
not maladapt, but does the best one can under the circumstances. Blame therefore is eliminated. The degree of health or equilibrium is determined by the
way a person copes with a particular set of circumstances and their duration
and toxicity. The set of circumstances can be called a *need, tension, force,
vector, strain, stress*, or *crisis*.

The well model promotes care of the whole person, as does nursing's ideal.
The total person is not just the sum of his or her parts, but is a singular, unique
being. The person does not just possess a brain, a family, and a home. All
aspects of a person's life space (the person and the total environment) become
integrated to become that particular individual. This is the reason focus on a
particular disease or a particular method of treatment, for example, behavioral
modification, neglects the concept of person.

With its broad frame of reference, the well model can also be adapted to
the nursing of other than dying clients. Both hospital- and non–hospital-based
nursing can use this model. Based on nursing care given in both episodic and
distributive settings, the model therefore will be useful in nursing's future, as
seen by the National Commission for the Study of Nursing and Nursing
Education:

> 1   One career pattern (episodic) would emphasize practice that is essentially

---

[1]R. Butler, *Social Functioning Framework: An Approach to the Human Behavior and Social
Environment Sequence*, New York, Council on Social Work Education, 1970, p. 20.

curative and restorative, generally acute or chronic in nature, and most frequently provided in the setting of the hospital and the in-patient facility.

    2 The second career pattern (distributive) would emphasize the nursing practice that is essentially designed for health maintenance and disease prevention, this is generally continuous in nature, seldom acute, and increasingly will take place in emergent institutional settings.[1]

In addition, all other health care personnel, when using the well model, can truly say that they belong to the health care, instead of the sickness care, professions. If newer forms of therapy allow for a view of the total person, the well model will be adaptable. On an even broader base, the model might be adaptable to other cultural or different sets of norms.

The application of the well model is limited by time. It is not adaptable to very rapid, functional, or part-task nursing care given to large numbers of clients. In this situation there is no time to consider the person.

Simply, the well model is not a formula but a way of thinking and treating. It is meant to be a description of the relationship of stressors and the ability of the person to meet these stressors.

Graphically the well model can be explained by modifying Lewin's field theory (Figure 3-4). The solid horizontal line is the current situation, assuming to be in approximate balance or equilibrium. After an analysis is made of all the variables impinging on the current situational line, the solid line may be adjusted or unfrozen (downward or upward) relative to the margin of equilibrium safety line. This adjustment is called *unfreezing and refreezing*. The slashed horizontal lines are the margins of equilibrium safety. Beyond these lines disequilibrium and disorganization may occur. Beyond these margins of equilibrium safety, crisis-intervention techniques may be needed.

Potentials are any factors affecting the current situation. The word *potential* refers to negative or problem aspects of a situation as well as to positive aspects, because there is a potential for growth. To determine whether a potential is negative or positive, answer the following question: In what direction would the line be moved if the potential was operating alone? Negative potentials can be moved to positive forces.

An analogy to crisis theory is appropriate here. Crisis theory, in treating a severe problem situation, seeks at least to restore the client to pre crisis level and at most to improve the precrisis level of adjustment by teaching better problem-solving behaviors. For instance, lack of hospitalization insurance can increase anxiety in the hospitalized person. Inadequate finances are a negative potential, increasing tension within the system. A social worker, finding alternate emergency financing, will move the potential to the positive side of the equilibrium line.

The arrows above the solid horizontal line and pointing downward are, in Lewin's words, *driving forces*. I prefer to call them *positive potentials*. These

[1]The National Commission for the Study of Nursing and Nursing Education: *An Abstract for Action*, New York, McGraw-Hill Book Co., 1970, pp. 91–92.

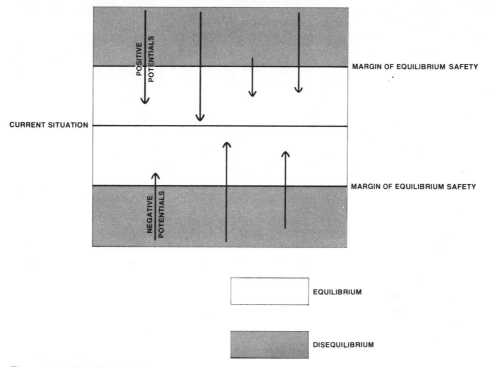

Figure 3-4   Modified field theory diagram of the well model.

are integration, a feeling of self-esteem, and physiological wholeness, in other words, support systems. Lewin attempts to quantify driving forces. I believe that at least in this situation and at the current state of knowledge in behavioral sciences, they cannot be quantified as yet. The word *potentials* is used in preference to driving forces because all these aspects of the person are potentially useful in current or future situations to maintain equilibrium and growth. Driving forces, and therefore potentials, keep the system moving. The arrows point downward representing the forces' effect on the current situation. Positive potentials are useful to manipulate in attempting to move the current situation line upward, but should not be used in isolation. By increasing the effect of positive potentials and not decreasing the effect of the restraining forces or negative potentials, tension within the system is increased.

. The arrows below the solid horizontal line and pointing upward are, in Lewin's words, *restraining forces*. Here they will be called *negative potentials*. These are aspects of a person's life space currently detracting from maintaining integration, a feeling of self-esteem, and physiological wholeness. Negative potentials have a direct effect on the current situation and influence the future situation. But these negative potentials may be moved to the positive side of the diagram by direct intervention, that is, by removing or decreasing certain factors, thereby bringing the person into a different state of equilibrium. Maslow might call them *deficiency needs* and claim that they retard movement. But negative potentials can be growth-producing.

As with the word *crisis*, negative potential also has aspects of both danger and opportunity. In addition, use of the words *negative potentials* is consistent with assumption 5, which states that "learning increases a person's strengths or potentials." Without the counterbalancing force of sufficient positive potentials, negative potentials may lead directly to disintegration. The restraining forces, or negative potentials, also cannot be quantified as yet.

Positive potentials such as close family ties can become negative if the family's inability to visit causes increased worry on the part of the client. To manipulate this potential, a provision for increasing visiting hours for the family or installation of a bedside phone may alleviate the anxiety.

The Need for Change

To implement care according to the well model, one must determine whether or not the need for change exists. By analyzing the current situation, the nurse may discover that the client is functioning adequately and little or no intervention is necessary. An adequate state of equilibrium may be maintained during illness.

The following two situations will illustrate assessing the need for change. They should be considered as examples of the variety of situations in which the need for change must be precisely and clearly identified before intervention can take place.

A child recovering from a tonsillectomy may be in an adequate state of equilibrium, especially since the parent is staying in the room giving nursing care. The relationship of the nurse to the child is indirect, while the relationship of the nurse to the parent is that of consultant, an observer making suggestions for care based on a medical treatment plan. The nurse's minimal involvement actually may enhance the healing process. With the parent in the room, instead of the nurse, who is a stranger, the child may cry less and therefore decrease the bleeding that can occur due to the stress of crying. The child is not a tonsillectomy but a child who has a temporary problem, tonsillectomy. She is normally healthy and functions as part of a family structure. Even small children have rights, and the human right to be comforted by her parent is being recognized. This child is reacting totally to the situation. In this situation the child may have a diagram like the one in Figure 3-5.

These potentials could change, creating a different situation. If the minimal bleeding were to increase, the positive potential would move to the negative side. If the parent were removed from the situation, even temporarily, the negative effect of the strange environment would intensify.

Recognition of the need for change is determined by a perception of violations of established norms. These are culturally and statistically determined standards. Physiologically, the established norm of, in the above situation, minimal bleeding, might be violated by increased bleeding. Sociologically, it is acceptable and preferred that the parent assume the role of primary provider of comfort and care.

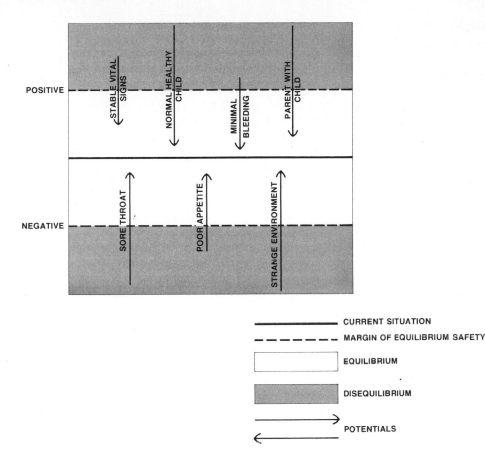

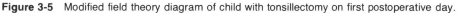

Figure 3-5   Modified field theory diagram of child with tonsillectomy on first postoperative day.

If the need for change is established, most likely the current situation line needs to be moved down. A problem can be identified before or after analysis of the current situation. The perception of a problem may be the reason to diagram a situation for further clarification.

When the need for change has been established, one must choose the most readily available potentials to manipulate; for instance, if the client's biggest problem is pain, this may often be readily relieved by medication. Then the equilibrium line can be unfrozen and moved down, indicating a different degree of equilibrium. With pain relief comes increased mobilization, active participation in the environment, and generally a less stressful situation.

Attempting to manipulate potentials is a two-step process. First, list all positive and negative potentials affecting the situation. Second, find the most accessible, or easiest, and most feasible, or practical, potentials to manipulate. The most accessible may not be the most feasible potentials. Trial and error may be necessary.

An example will clarify accessible but unfeasible potentials. A very common, complex situation involves a severely arteriosclerotic, geriatric, nonhospitalized client, for example, a grandfather. He prizes his independence yet seems unable to care for himself. His family, with whom he used to enjoy visiting, now wants to put him in a nursing home. His family feels that (1) he is irrational, irascible, unpredictable, and a potential danger to himself, (2) he refuses to have a housekeeper, and (3) all family members work and cannot care for him. Even if a family member could afford to care for him, the emotional burden of his full-time care would be too great. Moreover, the family has guilt feelings about wanting him in a nursing home.

In the above situation, the real problem is finding the most accessible, or easiest, and feasible, or practical, potentials to manipulate. A nursing home may be accessible in terms of location and finances, but the client's refusal to enter it makes it unfeasible. As time progresses, tension increases as the degree of deterioration of the elder person increases. With increasing conflict, the stability of the family structure is jeopardized. There are four possibilities that might occur without intervention. One, he remains home and falls, breaking his hip and precipitating immediate hospitalization. Two, he burns the house down accidentally from a lighted stove and, if he survives the fire, is hospitalized for burns. Three, he dies in his sleep. Four, irrational behavior forces the family to put him in a nursing home over the client's objection. This fourth possibility brings up a serious question of violation of client's rights. Only through legal channels can a family declare a member incompetent and have the person institutionalized.

Clearly this is an unstable situation, and without proper intervention and client cooperation, negative potentials—the client's confusion, irritational behavior, and deteriorating physical condition—will overcome his positive potentials—financial security and a caring, supportive family. There are no easy answers. All the limited possible solutions take time. First, and most drastically, the family could have him declared legally incompetent and for his safety's sake put him in a nursing home. This course of action may ruin or at least place a severe strain on family cohesiveness. To take someone's freedom away legally is a drastic and most distasteful step. The easiest solution is for the nurse and family to convince the client that he needs someone to live with him in his own house, for without close watching, accident, fire, or death is inevitable. Convincing the client may require promising him that the person who will move in will not interfere with his freedom but will only help him by being a companion.

It is always possible that the client, family, and nurse do not see the same solution as feasible. Change, then, toward a mutually desirable goal is impeded. For instance, the family may be blocked from making a decision by a view of nursing homes as a place for someone to be put away or die. The nurse's major concern may be for the grandfather's safety. To overcome this obstacle, the nurse can go with the family to visit a nursing home that provides quality care, or another health team member, such as a social worker or a psychologist, might have some suggestions for alternative action.

After analysis of the current situation and before nursing care can be implemented and change affected, a clear understanding of the desirab₁ᵣ rection of change is necessary. To maintain equilibrium, there often must be decreased tension in the system and conflict resolution to increase functioning and self-esteem.

Goal Setting

The modified field theory, or well model, cannot be used unless short-and long-term mutual goals are developed by all participants: client, family, professionals, and nonprofessionals. A clearer view of the situation can be obtained with the inclusion of the varying perspectives of a group of people. In addition, since all members are consulted and each person's view is considered important, everyone is more likely to strive toward the common goal. In a potentially curative situation, more rapid progress can be made toward recovery in this manner.

The client must take a responsible and active role in goal development. Only with mutual goal setting and understanding will he or she have reason to cooperate with the plan of care. The well model implies mutual trust of the helpers and client; coercion is eliminated. The passively submitting client is the coerced patient.

In the dying situation, a clearer understanding of client's, family's, and health care worker's mutually dependent roles is maintained. All involved may develop a sense of satisfaction. This implies the open awareness context of Glaser and Strauss, in which all communicants have acknowledged the forth-coming death and are able to discuss feelings openly. There are no ambiguities or concealment. Everyone works toward mutually agreed-upon goals. Most of all, the client does not experience feelings of abandonment. The goal of open communication can be set aside because of the myriad of complicated treatment modalities that are available. It is important that neither the client nor the person's goals get lost in the treatment plan.

Values

Goal setting occurs within the context of conscious and unconscious under-standing of subtle values, beliefs, and attitudes that have a significant impact on the modification of behavior. Force field theory is a theory of change in that it describes a process. Within that process values are the catalysts or forces that influence choices. The well model, as modified force field theory, is also a theory of change and is influenced by values. "A value is a conception, explicit or implicit, distinctive of an individual or characteristic of a group, of the desirable which influences the selection from available modes, means, and ends of action."[1] What is good is desirable, and what is bad is undesirable and to be eliminated. Because values are so deeply imbedded in a person, their role in behavior is not fully acknowledged. A person who is racially prejudiced

---

[1]C. Kluckhohn et al., "Values and Value-Orientations in the Theory of Action, An Exploration in Definition and Classification," in Parsons, T., and Shils, E. (eds.), *Toward a General Theory of Action*, Cambridge, Mass.: Harvard University Press, 1952, p. 395.

genuinely believes in the superiority of a particular race or creed. To others he or she is prejudiced, but to that individual the belief is morally justified or even factual.

The nurse and the client may not have the same values. Abortion is against many nurses' values. The woman seeking an abortion may be the object of unspoken disapproval. The abortion client, for instance, who receives minimal attention by nurses may be receiving tacit disapproval. This is a situation in which the law is clearly in conflict with the value systems of the nurses.

On the other hand, values of nurses and clients may be very similar. The reader would probably agree that nurses like their clients to have the characteristics stated in the following quotation. This study was conducted in 1962, but even with changes such as the growth of the patient's rights movement, these values and subsequent role behaviors still exist:

> Sixty-eight percent of the patients in the sample mentioned that they had refrained from expressing their desires, fears, or criticisms. When explaining this reluctance, the majority stressed the obligation of a patient over and above the privileges of a paying consumer and over and above the prerogatives of a sick person. The emphasis of these patients was on self-control, on a minimum of dependency, on being "cooperative," "undemanding," and "considerate." Patients were eager to cite instances confirming their adherence to these standards. When they were asked to describe themselves on an attribute scale they were guided by the desire to appear to others as "good" patients. They saw themselves as grateful, confident, trusting, cooperative, considerate, and undemanding.[1]

Mutual awareness of the system's norms and attempts on the part of both sides of an interaction not to violate these norms give implicit approval to behaviors necessary for care. Since health is a universally accepted value, efforts on the part of health care workers to restore it are usually met with approval. Moreover, health becomes more highly prized during illness.

As part of our value system we make prejudgments, deciding on the value or outcome of a situation before it occurs. The way we generalize has an effect on our prejudgments. Generalizing seems to make the complicated simpler, but often in generalizing we lose important individual qualities. For instance, by assuming no one wants to die alone, we do not consider someone who prefers to be alone in death. We may not even give a person a chance to express this wish. Also, stereotypical behaviors and attitudes are very difficult to root out once they are accepted as factual.

By constantly trying to make themselves more consciously aware of their values, beliefs, and attitudes, nurses can be more therapeutic. Nurses should understand that they cannot be therapeutic when personal values conflict with those of a client. On the basis of value conflict, nurses should ask another person not in conflict to assume the therapeutic role. On the other hand, nurses'

---

[1]D. Tagliacozzo, "The Nurse from the Patient's Point of View," in Skipper, J., and Leonard, R. (eds.), *Social Interaction and Patient Care*, Philadelphia, J. B. Lippincott Co., 1965, p. 222.

willingness to work with conflicting values by trying to understand the other person's values can be growth-producing.

The motto "know thyself " is important in the development of sensitivity to the client's needs. Along with a professional education, personal education is necessary. A conscientious, continuing effort toward clarification of personal values, beliefs, and attitudes would increase a nurse's understanding of his or her value system. Then there would be a basis for comparison with the client's value system. If nurses find they are not in harmony with their clients' views, they cannot assume that the clients are wrong or right.

Clients' Rights

Clients not only have the option to accept or refuse care, they also have the right and responsibility to determine the kind of treatment they will receive. Together, health care workers and clients assess acceptable modifications in life-style and plan and execute care.

The well model demands that nurses be ever vigilant of clients' rights, both legal and moral. An important part of the consumer revolution in health care was the effort of the American Hospital Association in 1973 to formalize clients' rights. Unfortunately, the organization "couched every statement in carefully guarded terms and avoided mention of certain topics that were sure to irritate the medical profession."[1]

Generally the hospital client's Bill of Rights that is used is a further modification of the originally watered-down American Hospital Association document. Moreover, whether the document is from the American Hospital Association or is a derivative of it, it is, in its entirety, only a set of guiding principles and not legal rights. We still have a long way to go to completely permit clients their rights. The particular legal rights, for example, the client's right to his or her own record, vary in each state, but acknowledged human rights are based on the prevailing value system. The clients' rights listed by Denenberg (see Appendix A) serve as more comprehensive guiding principles and further clarify the responsibilities of the health care system in providing high-quality care. Annas, too, provides a model Bill of Rights. If the reader's hospital has a Bill of Rights it would be enlightening to compare it with the Denenberg and Annas documents.

In a definite step forward, the federal government supports the client's right to chart accessibility:

> The Commission [of the Department of Health, Education and Welfare on Medical Malpractice] FINDS that patients have a right to the information contained in their medical records and RECOMMENDS that such information be made more easily accessible to patients, and the Commission further RECOMMENDS that the States enact legislation enabling patients to obtain access to the information contained in their medical records through their legal representatives, public or private, without having to file suit.

[1]N. Quinn and A. Somers, "The Patient's Bill of Rights, A Significant Aspect of the Consumer Revolution," *Nursing Outlook*, 22(2):242, April 1974.

The Commission [of the Department of Health, Education and Welfare on Medical Malpractice] RECOMMENDS that the States enact legislation to prohibit modification alteration or destruction of medical records with the intent of misleading or misinforming patients.[1]

Eight states allow clients direct access to their own records; they are Illinois, Connecticut, New Jersey, Massachusetts, Wisconsin, Oklahoma, Virginia, and Colorado. Two states allow a client access to records through an attorney. This latter process, of course, is time-consuming and expensive and therefore discriminatory against the poorest clients. The rationale behind it is that it allows the attorney to be a screening agent, thereby ensuring that the client's best interests are served. Attorneys are no more knowledgeable about medicine than other lay people. Mississippi requires good reason for release of records to the client. In Virginia a written statement from the physician stating that information in the record would be injurious to the client can prevent the client from seeing the record. Laws governing client access to medical records do not include psychiatric records. They are generally not available to clients.

The arguments against allowing clients direct access to their charts have many proponents. Clients could misinterpret what is written. For instance, in the diagnostic process cancer is often considered. Even though cancer might be eliminated as a diagnosis, the client, seeing the word on the chart, might be unduly upset. What, though, prevents a physician from explaining that cancer was eliminated and revealing the actual diagnosis? Also, clients who do not understand the language in the chart could have someone translate it and answer questions.

At the heart of the argument over chart accessibility is the issue of physician and hospital accountability. If the client could see the chart, the physician and hospital obviously would be more accountable for any errors in judgment and practice. This is truly a volatile issue, because physicians and all the hospitals' staffs can make mistakes.

However, there is more to client's rights than legislation. The interpersonal issue of privacy is a privilege and a right that when overlooked diminishes a person's dignity and autonomy:

> The development and maintenance of individuality have been related to the need for autonomy. Some behavioral scientists have described interpersonal relationships in terms of zones, regions, or circles of privacy leading to the core of the inner self. The inner portion contains those secrets, thoughts, and beliefs which are not shared with anyone except in situations of extreme stress when the person must share of essential emotional relief.[2]

[1]U.S. Department of Health, Education and Welfare, *Medical Malpractice, Report of the Secretary's Commission on Medical Malpractice*, Washington, D.C., U.S. Government Printing Office, January 16, 1973, p. 77.

[2]D. Bloch, "Privacy," in Carlson, C. (ed.), *Behavioral Concepts and Nursing Intervention*, Philadelphia, J. B. Lippincott Co., 1970, p. 253.

Privacy can be welcome solitude or dreaded isolation. Absolute privacy for prolonged periods of time, the effects of which are sometimes called *sensory deprivation*, can be disastrous for both human and animal. However, a sense of territoriality and privacy of space is essential to survival for humans and many animals. Essentially, with the cooperation and respect of the larger group, an individual needs to maintain control over time, place, manner, and amount of information revealed about himself or herself. The need to withhold information or maintain social distance may be met through physical means such as closing of a door, or through psychological means, such as mode of attire or speech. The client is entitled to privacy and the nurse can be the advocate who helps maintain that privacy.

Client Advocacy

The role of the client advocate is emerging. Various types of people have been used in client advocate roles: students of various professions, paramedics trained in medical ethics, and sensitive volunteers. Some hospitals have hired people with the job title *ombudsman* or *advocate* to serve as liaison between client and health care workers. They may actually become all-purpose complaint departments or, because hired by the hospital, take on a public relations role.

For years there have been protests against the increasing fragmentation of care in the sickness care professions. The employment of a specially designated advocate may complicate the situation in that there is one more person with whom to interact in an already overcrowded hierarchy of people. But the advocate may be a necessary intermediary step as the consumer becomes increasingly informed. The solution to the advocacy problem is for the clients themselves to become aware of their rights and insist on exercising them.

As the persons most frequently in contact, nurses must try to inform clients. They must avoid using medical terminology that confuses clients. They must relinquish some of the decision making to the clients. They must be willing to work cooperatively *with* and not *on* the clients.

In terms of the overall power structure of the hospital and the sickness care system, nurses must learn a more sophisticated use of power. As persons hired by the hospital and the sickness care system, they have a potential conflict of interest. In any situation, to whom are they accountable? Certainly they are accountable to the clients, but to what degree must the norms and prevailing value system of the hospital and the sickness care system be followed? This is sometimes a difficult question to answer, but in reality, much more could be done by nurses in their role as advocates than is already currently being accomplished.

For those clients unable to make decisions, safeguards to preserve the quality of life must be established. The senile, retarded, and mentally ill, for example, involuntarily relinquish choices in their care. Even if they do have the ability to speak, they may not be able to give informed consent. Thus, such crucial decisions as potential for self-care must be made by someone else. If it is determined that self-care is not feasible, the alternatives—who, where, and when the client will be cared for—must be made by someone else. Who is the best qualified person to decide? Is there a conflict of interest that may sway a decision? Surely those unable to give informed consent need an advocate.

SUMMARY

The archaic sick model, focusing on the passive patient who is the recipient of care, needs to be replaced by the well model, which focuses on the client as an active participant in treatment, having rights and responsibilities as a human being. All clients have some strengths and coping abilities that should be used to help them withstand the stress of illness.

The well model is defined in terms of the dynamics of health, stress, adaptation, equilibrium, margin of safety, and sickness as a continuum. Coping implies successful overcoming of a challenge, while adaptation is the unifying mechanism whereby the person flexibly integrates new experiences, unconsciously and consciously. Coping is successful adaptation. Maladaptation does not exist as it is usually defined, that is, as failure to adapt appropriately to stresses and therefore progression to disorganization and collapse. In extreme stress the client does not maladapt but adapts to the only choice he or she sees available, and that choice leads to disorganization and collapse.

Seven assumptions support the well model. They are as follows:

1   Human beings have a special uniqueness seen only when one observes their totality.
Viewing a person as the sum of parts obscures the relationship of parts to the whole person. Many ideas, for instance, love, hate, pain, crisis, and stress, can be viewed only in their totality.
2   The natural tendency of each person is toward at least survival and at most health and equilibrium.
Free will and motivation are the keys to meeting our survival drives. The belief in the value of and innate drive for survival must be the basis of the therapeutic process and relationship.
3   Wellness or health and, therefore, survival are dependent upon the ability of the person to adapt.
Genetic adaptation can be seen in Darwin's concept of evolution of species. The organism adapts physiologically to internal and environmental stresses according to the general or biological adaptation syndrome. Crisis theory is a model of psychological adaptation.
4   Each person is responsible for his or her own actions.
The United States Constitution, democracy, and subsequently the client's Bill of Rights are based on the individual's assuming responsibility.
5   Learning increases a person's strengths or potentials.
To enhance genetic endowment, each person learns to survive and fulfill himself or herself. From one's learning how to feed oneself to the client's learning self-care for a new diabetic condition, the goal is improvement.
6   Stress is normal and necessary for growth and development.

Stress is the effect of the body's initiating any adaptive change. It is necessary for self-fulfillment.

.7 Individuals adapt to stressors in different ways.
        •

Some of the endless variation in stress reactions results from the maturation level of the individual. Environmental supports can help a person adapt to stress. The well model is meant to be a description of the relationships of stressors and the ability of the person to meet these stressors.

Schematically it is adapted from Lewin's field theory. Each person possesses certain positive potentials, the strengths and coping abilities that help to maintain equilibrium. A person may have a problem, or a negative potential. Both positive and negative potentials impinge on the current situation, changing the level of equilibrium. The level of adaptation that eventually results in equilibrium is always changing. However, there is a margin of equilibrium safety beyond which the individual will disorganize and collapse.

Explicit in the well model is mutual goal setting between nurses, other health care professionals, and clients as an essential part of any decision-making process. The need for change must be determined within the framework of values.

The well model cannot be implemented unless nurses look at their value systems. It is especially important to do this when their values conflict with clients' and therefore their ability to be therapeutic is jeopardized. Trying to work through a conflict in value systems by nurse and client can be growth-producing.

Intrinsic in the well model is the need of the nurse to support the client's legal and moral rights. The client's Bill of Rights is a set of guiding principles that some states and many institutions have adapted to not only ensure clients' rights but also promote the increasing accountability of all health care professionals. In addition to legislated rights, other rights, such as personal privacy, need to be acknowledged and respected.

To ensure adequate implementation of these rights, the client needs an advocate. The nurse should act in this role. Some hospitals have hired client advocates to serve as liaison between clients and health care personnel. Those clients unable to give informed consent are in special need of an advocate. The advocate is only an intermediary to aid in informing the consumer. Clients ultimately need to be their own advocates.

The well model, useful in many areas of nursing, is especially useful in care of the dying. Subsequent chapters will illustrate the well model's use in care of the dying.

QUESTIONS FOR REFLECTION AND DISCUSSION

3-1 What does *health* mean to you? Ask five people of different cultures what *health* means to them. Compare the answers.

3-2   As a healthy person, what physical, emotional, and social stresses are you experiencing?

3-3   In what ways do you adapt to these stresses?

3-4   What support systems do you have in your life?

3-5   Diagram a client situation in terms of positive and negative potentials. Does the situation need intervention? If so, what potentials should be moved?

3-6   Choose a hospitalized client. What physical, emotional, and social stresses is he or she experiencing? How is the client adapting to these stresses? How are the person's developmental tasks being thwarted during hospitalization?

3-7   What kinds of adaptations to stresses can cause further stresses?

BIBLIOGRAPHY

Aguilera, D., and Messick, J.: *Crisis Intervention, Theory and Methodology*, St. Louis, C. V. Mosby Co., 1974.

Barrell, L.: "Crisis Intervention, Partnership in Problem Solving," *Nursing Clinics of North America* 9(1):5–16, March 1974.

Bloch, D.: "Privacy," in Carlson, C. E. (ed.), *Behavioral Concepts and Nursing Intervention*, Philadelphia, J. B. Lippincott Co., 1970.

Bronowski, J.: *The Ascent of Man*, Boston, Little, Brown and Co., 1973.

Butler, R.: *Social Functioning Framework: An Approach to the Human Behavior and Social Environment Sequence*, New York, Council on Social Work Education, 1973.

Chapple, E., and Coon, C.: *Principles of Anthropology*, New York, Henry Holt and Co., 1942.

Darwin, C.: *The Origin of Species*, New York, Everyman's Library, 1928.

Dubos, R.: *So Human an Animal*, New York, Charles Scribner's Sons, 1968.

————: *The Torch of Life*, New York, Simon & Schuster, 1962.

Fromm, E.: *Escape from Freedom*, New York, Holt, Rinehart and Winston, 1941.

Halstad, L.: "The Use of Crisis Intervention in Obstetrical Nursing," *The Nursing Clinics of North America*, 9(1):69–76, March 1974.

Hospital Law Manual, Administrator's Volume, vol. IA, Health Law Center, Aspen Systems Corp.

Hospital Law Manual, Attorney's Volume, vol. IIA, Health Law Center, Aspen Systems Corp., 1977.

Hardy, M. (ed.): *Theoretical Foundations for Nursing*, New York, MSS Information Corp., 1973.

King, I.: *Toward a Theory for Nursing*, New York, John Wiley and Sons, 1971.

Kluckhohn, C., et al.: "Values and Value-Orientation in the Theory of Action, An Exploration in Definition and Classification," in Parsons, T., and Shils, E. (eds.), *Toward a General Theory of Action*, Cambridge, Mass., Harvard University Press, 1952.

Kramer, M.: *Reality Shock*, St. Louis, C. V. Mosby Co., 1974.

Levine, S., and Scotch, N. (eds.): *Social Stress*, Chicago, Aldine Publishing Co., 1970.

Lewin, K.: *A Dynamic Theory of Personality*, New York, McGraw-Hill Book Co., 1935.

————: *Field Theory in Social Science*, New York, Harper and Brothers, 1951.

Lindemann, C.: "Influencing Recovery through Preoperative Teaching," *Heart and Lung, The Journal of Critical Care*, 2(4):515–521, 1973.

Maslow, A.: *Toward a Psychology of Being*, New York, D. Van Nostrand Co., 1968.

Moustakis, C.: *Creativity and Conformity*, New York, D. Van Nostrand Co., 1967.

The National Commission for the Study of Nursing and Nursing Education: *An Abstract for Action*, New York, McGraw-Hill Book Co., 1970.

Oklahoma Session Law Service, chaps. 21–60, 36th legislature, convened January 4, 1977, St. Paul, Minn., West Publishing Co.

Parsons, T.: *The Social System*, New York, Free Press, 1951.

Power, E.: *Evaluation of Educational Doctrine: Major Educational Theorists of the Western World*, New York, Appleton-Century-Crofts, 1969.

Quinn, N., and Somers, A.: "The Patient's Bill of Rights; A Significant Aspect of the Consumer Revolution," *Nursing Outlook*, **22**(2):240–244, April 1974.

Rapoport, R.: "The State of Crisis: Some Theoretical Considerations," in Parad, H. (ed.), *Crisis Intervention: Selected Readings*, New York, Family Service Association of America, 1965.

Read, P.: *Alive, the Story of the Andes Survivors*, Philadelphia, J. B. Lippincott Co., 1974.

Rogers, C.: *On Becoming a Person*, Boston, Houghton Mifflin Co., 1961.

Rogers, M.: *An Introduction to the Theoretical Basis of Nursing*, Philadelphia, F. A. Davis Co., 1970.

Russett, C.: *The Concept of Equilibrium Theory in American Social Thought*, New Haven, Conn., Yale University Press, 1966.

Selye, H.: *Stress without Distress*, Philadelphia, J. B. Lippincott Co., 1974.

————: *The Stress of Life*, New York, McGraw-Hill Book Co., 1956.

Smith, D.: "*Patienthood and Its Threat to Privacy*," *American Journal of Nursing*, **69**(3): 509–513, March 1969.

Tagliacozzo, D.: "The Nurse from the Patient's Point of View," in Skipper, J., and Leonard, R. (eds.), *Social Interaction and Patient Care*, Philadelphia, J. B. Lippincott Co., 1965.

Toffler, A.: *Future Shock*, New York, Random House, 1970.

U.S. Department of Health, Education and Welfare: *Medical Malpractice, Report of the Secretary's Commission on Medical Malpractice*, Washington D.C., U.S. Government Printing Office, January 16, 1973.

Wu, R.: *Behavior and Illness*, Engelwood Cliffs, N.J., Prentice-Hall, 1973.

Chapter 4

The Well Model Applied to the Nursing Process

Although the well model has applicability in all health care professions, in this chapter it will be applied to the nursing process to aid nurses in their flexible and changing role expectations of today and tomorrow. All phases of the nursing process will be identified and discussed briefly, but major emphasis will be on assessment and the strength-oriented nursing record. The positive potentials (strengths) and negative potentials (problems) are related to acutely and chronically dying clients in later chapters.

In recent years nursing activities have been systematized into a multistep process, similar to the steps of the problem-solving process. The value of this approach lies in its clearly organizing the same activities nurses have traditionally performed and leading the way to identification of the future expanded roles of the nurse, such as that of the independent practitioner. Various authors have described the nursing process in three to six steps. As long as all relevant aspects are implicitly included, the number of steps or substeps identified is arbitrary. Since nursing is a *process*, steps sometimes overlap and blur to the point where an activity takes on all aspects of the process, as in teaching colostomy care. While assessing a client's needs and ability to learn, the therapist may also be cleaning the colostomy and evaluating the condition around the stoma and the client's reaction to the colostomy. Therefore, *the nursing process* is a general term for a planned therapeutic interaction of nurse and client intended to maintain or return the client to a state of maximum well-being.

COMPLEMENTARY NATURE OF WELL MODEL AND NURSING PROCESS

Both the nursing process and the well model view the client from a unitary or integrated perspective and from an advocacy focus. Both are also goal-directed. The well model nursing process retains the usual steps: (1) assessment, (2) planning, (3) intervention, and (4) evaluation, but it emphasizes growth rather than maintenance, plus the rights and responsibilities of the giver and receiver of care and mutual goal setting:

> The nursing process is basically set up for one purpose: to encourage the nurse to use a problem-solving approach in assisting the patient to understand his life process or style so that he can better control and cope with his illness (and make the most of his wellness).*

The well model views the client as a person with rights and responsibilities, functioning in the real world in a relative state of equilibrium on the health-illness continuum. The degree of equilibrium is dependent upon the balance of positive and negative potentials the person has for meeting life's situations. Stress is an ever-present phenomenon to which the person reacts with positive and negative potentials. Focus on strengths, coping, and problem-solving abilities provides a broader analysis of problems. So much has been written about problem identification; I feel it is unnecessary to duplicate the literature. The more pressing need is for exhaustive research on factors involved in the coping process.

USE IN DISTRIBUTIVE AND EPISODIC SETTINGS

The broad well model nursing process goal, that is, maintaining maximum well-being, is implemented in a variety of settings, but the specific actions differ. Nurses' professional goals are dependent upon their psychological and physical makeup, internalized view of their role, external forces such as institutional policy, and previous experience.

In a distributive setting, that is, an outclient facility such as a primary care clinic, the aim is health maintenance and disease prevention. Here the client will probably present mostly positive potentials. Nursing care emphasizes identifying and recording coping mechanisms for current and future use and health teaching. As different health care workers care for the client, a record of not only a client's problem but also coping patterns and abilities accumulates and is available for reference.

*S. Carlson, "A Practical Approach to the Nursing Process," *American Journal of Nursing*, **72**(9):1591, September 1972.

In an episodic setting, that is, an institutional or inclient facility, the well model nursing process is more easily seen. The client enters the episodic setting for acute or chronic curative or rehabilitative care even though he or she may be dying. Problems are assumed because the client has a disease process or at least symptoms of a dysfunction. The nurse using the well model nursing process would see both the client's illness-related problems and his or her coping strengths. In both distributive and episodic settings, the nurse can use the well model nursing process in independent practice or as part of a health care team.

EVALUATION OF THE PROBLEM-ORIENTED RECORD

Nursing has widely adapted the problem-oriented record (POR). As a recording system it effectively simplifies and standardizes complex data. It is also an instrument for establishing quality control through periodic auditing by the individual and team members. Information in the POR is readily fed into computers to accumulate a rich source of research material. In the education of nurses, the POR is focused not on memory learning but more appropriately on teaching adaptable behavioral changes that are both analytically sound and efficient. Nursing might use the POR as readily available documentation in licensure and related issues, such as accountability, peer review, professional certification, and continued competency.

The POR follows the basic problem-solving steps. One, it contains a data base developed from history, physical data, and admission laboratory data. Two, a complete list of problems, both active and inactive, is extracted from the data base. Three, future plans for treating and resolving each problem are elaborated along with the collection of further data, treatment, and client education. Four, chronological and sequential progress notes are accumulated.

But the POR has problems. Developed by a physician, the POR includes all elements of the sick model. The physician assesses and treats the patient's problems. No effort is made at mutual goal setting or maintaining client privacy. Weed in fact makes no mention of any client's legal or human rights but rather stresses the POR as an educational and research tool.

The major advantage of the POR, that of a clearly identifiable data base, has been misused. This misuse centers around the definition of *problem*. Since nursing and medicine can traditionally see only problems, the POR creates problems where none exist. For example, Bonkowsky uses the POR in community child health care. She lists "routine health supervision" as a problem. Routine health supervision is not a problem, and it becomes a problem only if an obstacle, such as an inability to understand health teaching, is present. Because a problem is not found, this does not render the nursing process purposeless and functionless. Maintaining maximum well-being also includes reinforcing the client's positive potentials. Moreover, the POR has been most effective in identifying physical problems, while psychological or social problems are addressed in vague terms. They need to be specified with criteria and performance standards.

The POR is just another instance of how nursing uses what has been developed in medicine. Nursing should be able to develop independent methods and functions compatible with those of medicine. Nurses have something unique to offer health care. That elusive goal—total client care—can become a reality, but not until the client's strengths are at least acknowledged. The proposed strength-oriented nursing record, which follows, is a means of identifying a client's strengths. The problem in devising this record is that a unified theory of how people cope does not exist.

REVIEW OF STEPS IN THE NURSING PROCESS

1   *Assessment*   To obtain as much data as possible about the client, the nurse's primary source of information is the client's history and physical examination. Supplementary sources of information may be old records, family, laboratory data, and other team members. Assessment culminates in a diagnosis.

2   *Planning*   To clarify problems, goals, strengths, actions, and expected behavioral outcomes, the nurse, team members, and client make decisions in terms of priorities that are short-, intermediate-, and long-term goals. Entering this information as specifically as possible into the nursing care plan is essential.

3   *Implementation*   Nursing actions may take the form of direct nursing care, such as administering treatments and medications, or may take the form of interpersonal communication. A large part of the implementation phase concerns client education for coping today and in the future.

4   *Evaluation*   The nursing audit is one way to identify for the nurse and the client both the goals achieved and the needs met, in order to evaluate care. The client's strengths and how they were useful to client and nurse should also be included.

ASSESSMENT

The well model is most useful in the assessment process and in the first two parts of the problem-oriented record, the data base and the problem list. Problems or negative potentials can be identified, classified, analyzed, and summarized, and positive potentials, areas of strength, and coping mechanisms can be ascertained during the assessment.

The initial assessment, called a *nursing history* and obtained by a professional nurse, provides a baseline of facts and observations from which to view change over time. This baseline can be obtained by several methods.

First, using experience, observation, and communication skills, an interviewer elicits facts, attitudes, and behaviors pertinent to future nursing care. An interview provides a beginning opportunity to establish a trusting relationship.

Using inductive and deductive reasoning the nurse obtains information about the client. The nurse makes inferences about the client's appearance, behavior, and attitudes. These inferences need validation throughout the nursing process as more information is added to the assessment. To validate inferences, for instance, clarifying questions may be asked. Validation by other team members may also be helpful in arriving at a precise assessment. Much more difficult to obtain than information about facts such as blood pressure or housing, and subject to easy misinterpretation, are questions about attitudes and understanding. In order to better evaluate nonverbal behavior, the nurse should think about the following questions:

1   What is the client's affect? Is it congruent with the words being spoken?
2   Does the affect change during the interview?
3   What is the client's posture? Is it rigid or relaxed?
4   What kinds of gestures does the client use with his or her head, hands, feet, or legs?

In addition, it is important to clarify the client's understanding of the illness. If, for example, the client states that the diagnosis was not disclosed, there are four possible explanations: (1) the client really was not told, (2) the client was told and did not hear, (3) the client was told, heard, and now is denying the diagnosis, or (4) the client was told and did not understand because of the technical language used in the explanation, a psychological block, or a hearing impairment. "The client himself becomes the connecting link between the decision-making process and the nursing process, and he is the determining factor for the successful interrelated use of both processes."*

Second, a review of the previous medical and nursing record will be informative in terms of former problems, methods used for coping, and previous strengths. If coping and other strengths are not explicitly defined, special care should be taken to explore these areas in the initial interview. The nurse, for instance, not only should ask about allergies to pain medication, but also should ask how the client coped with pain at home and during prior hospitalization. A complete pain history is also helpful. The client's usual coping behaviors should be made known to other nursing personnel.

A third method of obtaining initial information about a client is by asking other members of the health team who have formerly cared for the client. Although helpful in completing a picture of the client, views of other personnel may be shaded by previously developed biases. Prejudgments on this basis can be dangerous and may inhibit effective communication and care. Especially important, if the client is unable to give accurate information, is the family's knowledge of the client and the events leading to the current illness.

Additionally, a physical assessment may be part of the initial history-taking procedure. Several books on physical assessment are listed at the back of this chapter. Developing expertise in physical assessment requires much time and

*J. Schaefer, "The Interrelatedness of Decision-Making and the Nursing Process," *American Journal of Nursing*, **74**(10):1854, October 1974.

training, and the reading of a book must be combined with clinical experience under the supervision of a competent nurse practitioner and teacher.

An assessment tool or nursing history form would be helpful only if it were used to see the total person. The tool, in constant revision, would accommodate the continually increasing information about and the evolving needs of the client. As part of mutual goal setting the client would also be given a copy of the form.

On the other hand, there are some definite limitations in the use of assessment tools. An assessment form cannot be useful if it is an end in itself. Checklists then become formulas. "Care is made professional by the manner in which it is provided. Technical care is a task done as an end in itself; the same activity is made part of professional care when it becomes a means to an end."* A nurse can misuse an assessment form by seeing only a checklist of items to complete and thinking that with completion of these items everything pertinent is known about the client. In other words, the attitude might prevail that the situation has been fully developed and understood, but that is not the nursing *process*. The nurse must consider the human factors involved: changes in oneself and in the client over time, the possibility of interpretive error, and incompleteness of information gathering on one's part.

After data are collected, nurses' interpretation of findings, sometimes called a *nursing diagnosis*, leads to the development of goals, followed by the taking of appropriate actions. A nurse's interpretation of the client's problems, strengths, and coping behaviors must be validated with the client so mutually acceptable goals for care can be developed. As a partner in health care, the client then is willing to work with a plan of treatment and care. If the client is unable to verbalize effectively, other methods of validation are necessary, such as observation of nonverbal behavior, use of tactile and olfactory senses, diagnostic data, previous records, and consultation with other team members, including family, who know the client.

Most hospitals have a version of the nursing history assessment form, consisting of a series of questions about dentures, food, bowel and sleeping habits, vital signs, allergies, medications, and other personal and physical data. Usually included on this form are the nurse's observations of the client, for instance, alertness or distress and initial reaction to illness and hospitalization. Since several examples of nursing history forms have been presented in the literature, no attempt will be made here to develop a general multipurpose assessment tool.

THEORETICAL FRAMEWORK FOR THE STRENGTH-ORIENTED NURSING RECORD

Assumptions

1   Stress is an inevitable part of living.

*N. Martin et al., "Nurses Who Nurse," *American Journal of Nursing*, 73(8):1384, August 1973.

2 Every person has a pattern of coping developed as a result of previous life experiences.

3 What is a crisis to one person may not be a crisis for another person, due to relative coping abilities.

4 As the degree of stress intensifies, the coping responses become more primitive.

According to the literature, there is no organized, generally accepted theory of coping, just as there is no generally accepted theory or even generally accepted definition of stress. Every person develops useful coping behaviors under stressful circumstances. Some behaviors are productive in that they lead to mastery and growth, and some eventually are destructive and lead to disintegration. Some people seem to have a better ability to function under stress than others do. Bruner calls that overall ability to adapt to life experiences with growth *integrity of functioning*. Phillips calls that adaptive potential the *achieved level of psychological development*, including intellectual, social, and moral spheres.

It is very difficult to differentiate coping mechanisms other than to state that coping that appears to help maintain equilibrium is good and that which leads to disorganization is bad. Defining good and bad coping becomes a problem of values, times, and cultures. Brunner defines coping as a process that

> respects the requirements of problems we encounter while still respecting our integrity. Defending is a strategy whose objective is avoiding or escaping from problems for which we believe there is no solution that does not violate our integrity of functioning . . . neither coping nor defending is found often in pure forms.*

Although patterns of coping can be identified, the variables operative in meeting stressful situations are almost infinite.

The normal healthy body provides the essential foundation for coping. In contrast, the physically ill person is more vulnerable to other stresses. Genetic endowment provides the building blocks for future development of coping behaviors. The mentally retarded, for instance, seem to have less ability to solve problems and cope with change, are less mature for a given age, and have fewer opportunities for social encounters from which to learn new coping behaviors.

Developmentally, a person learns to cope in large part by trial and error. If one method of attempting to alleviate discomfort does not work, another is tried until relief is attained.

Ethnic, socioeconomic, and religious variables play a major role in coping. As part of the fiber of a person, culture provides a rich source of learned and acceptable behavior patterns. Under stress each nationality allows certain ways

*J. Bruner, *Toward a Theory of Instruction*, Cambridge, Mass., The Belknap Press of Harvard University Press, 1966, pp. 129–30.

of handling emotions. Generalizations are often made about, for example, the stoicism of the Chinese or the verbalism of Latins in regard to pain response. The stereotypical Anglo-Saxon response to death is one of reserve or quiet acceptance. Control of one's feelings is typically both an Anglo-Saxon and a middle-class value. In addition, religious beliefs and ritual may have a calming and stabilizing effect on the ill client. It is necessary to understand that acceptable cultural patterns of behavior and attitude do exist but not to lose sight of the individual differences.

Although culture is significant in developing coping patterns, Lazarus has identified culture-free internal and external conditions for coping ability. Cognitive appraisal, that is, knowledge of some discomfort, is necessary to activate coping response. The person in the prodromal, undiagnosed, asymptomatic part of a terminal illness does not experience the psychological stress of illness, does not feel threatened, and therefore does not initiate coping processes.

Actual coping depends also upon several other factors, not the least of which is the accuracy or distortion of the real impact of the threat. It is here that defense mechanisms, which "are psychological maneuvers in which the individual deceives himself about the actual condition of threat,"* help maintain equilibrium temporarily or actually prevent adequate coping from taking place. Defense mechanisms falsify reality whereas coping mechanisms are task- and reality-oriented.

In addition, four variables affect coping ability. One is intensity of the threat. A threat becomes more intense if an important goal is thwarted. In any case, the intensity of the threat determines motivation for coping and actual coping ability. A client with a lump in her breast feels intensely threatened because of the possibility of (1) fatal illness and (2) damage to her body image and sexuality. Strong coping behaviors must be mobilized to meet this threat.

Two, the immediacy of the danger or the location of the agent of harm determines the choice of coping maneuvers. If a person can see no immediate danger in unhealthy living patterns, he or she will not be motivated to change them. Smoking may be given up only after a person has experienced the first heart attack or after an x-ray has shown a lung lesion.

Three, the inability to find alternative actions is also a significant determinant of coping behaviors. The person who sees no means of escape, for instance from a prison, becomes passive, but the person with one available escape route uses all available energy to effect the escape. Or, the dying client may seek out every charlatan in the vain hope of finding a cure.

Four, social and situational constraints that may lead to harm prevent adequate coping. Because of strong moral convictions against killing, a person may be unable to defend himself or herself when being attacked.

Situational and developmental stresses make a person more vulnerable and require coping adaptation. Surgery, acute illness, and chronic illness make a person more vulnerable. Throughout the life cycle a person experiences tran-

*R. Lazarus, *Psychological Stress and the Coping Process*, New York, McGraw-Hill Book Co., 1966, p. 265.

sitional states, which Erikson calls *normative crisis* periods, requiring major changes in role behaviors and increasing a person's vulnerability to stress. A glance at Erikson's eight stages of man shows that it is "normal" for an older person to contemplate death as he or she sees contemporaries dying. But how are the 18-year-old's developmental tasks changed when facing death? Dying is in and of itself a very vulnerable state. The dying adolescent, experiencing both situational and developmental stresses, is extremely vulnerable and must cope with that vulnerability.

In summary, the nurse is concerned with the present and the future of clients. Care is given in the context of long-term goals. Inherent in these goals is an approximate appraisal of the person's ability to cope. If a person were completely devoid of coping strengths both psychological and physical, there could be no future for that person. All client education is predicated on (1) a presumed ability to learn and (2) an attempt to improve the person's future well-being, that is, improve ability to adapt to the exigencies of living, often with a chronic illness. Therefore, the nurse's accurate appraisal of the client's future adjustment to living and dying is essential to nursing care.

Assessment: The Key to the Strength-Oriented Nursing Record

Nurses usually are quite skillful at assessing problems, or negative potentials. Much has been written about clients' problems, but little attention has been given to the positive potentials of client care.

The strength-oriented nursing record (SONR) can be obtained in the same manner as the routine assessment of clients, that is, from client interviews, review of previous medical and nursing record, and input from other members of health care team and family members. Both subjective and objective data lend insight.

In addition, nurses must possess certain personal qualities and professional knowledge to ferret out a client's strengths. They must have an understanding of human behavior. They must take the time to become effective communicators with each client, thereby establishing a rapport. Their understanding of normal and abnormal psychology and physiology will help them decide whether a client is using growth-producing behavior and therefore is coping adequately. Knowledge of cultural mores and religious practices also will help nurses understand the appropriateness of coping behaviors in a particular client. Intuition is also helpful.

In addition, nurses' own subjective feelings about a client can have a marked effect on the interview and the subsequent therapeutic relationship. These feelings can cause distortion of the meaning of information received. For this reason validation of information by another team member is helpful. The following questions may help nurses to understand their reactions to a client:

1 What kinds of feelings does this client evoke in me? Anger? Sympathy?
2 How is the client responding to me?
3 As the client talks to me, what personal experiences am I reminded of?

The three major areas of emphasis in assessing clients' strengths are (1) systems review, (2) illness-related history, (3) social profile.

Systems Review

Physical assessment, or systems review, may reveal many areas of normalcy, for instance, vision, hearing, mobility, and speech, along with the chief complaint. *Normal* in a physical examination is usually referred to as *negative*, or without problem. Weed refers to *normal* euphemistically as having *significant negatives*, such as no blood in the urine.* Negatives, or "no problem" areas, once ascertained are then discarded. The sick model's focus on problems as good and normalcy as bad needs to be reversed. "Good" clients are very sick. The well model makes use of negatives or normal aspects of clients. Laboratory data also should be classified, when appropriate, as normal, not negative. Moreover, all these areas of normalcy may be used to ease the strain of sickness care.

Illness-Related History

Illness-related assessment includes present and past illnesses. Description of the present chief complaint should be followed by signs and symptoms, length of time experienced, and measures taken by client to help himself or herself, including medications.

The nurse can not only ascertain information about the illness, but also determine how it affects the client's daily life. The relationship of illness and stress should be considered by the nurse.

The answers to the following questions can help determine the appropriateness and the quality of the client's coping behaviors and possibly the need for teaching:

1 How is your physical health?
2 In what ways are you aware of your body right now?
3 What were the first symptoms you noticed?
4 Were you under some stress when your symptoms appeared?
5 What did you first do about these symptoms?
6 Did you try to handle things by yourself?
7 Did you ignore the symptoms?
8 Did you treat yourself or take any home remedies?
9 Have you sought other professional help?
10 Did you follow professional advice? If not, why not?
11 How did your family react to your health problems?
12 What are your goals for the treatment plan?

In eliciting illness-related information, the nurse is able to discover some areas of coping. A juvenile diabetic, for instance, who jogs when she feels weak

*L. Weed, *Medical Records, Medical Evaluation, and Patient Care; the Problem-Oriented Record as a Basic Tool*, Cleveland, Ohio, The Press of Case Western Reserve University, 1970, p. 24.

and thinks her blood sugar is elevated, displays nonproductive coping behaviors. The need for diabetic teaching appears to be obvious, but more covert problems may be at the root of the ineffective coping behavior. A nurse may be able to take this negative potential, or problem, and turn it into a positive potential useful for maintaining health and equilibrium.

On the other hand, a person with angina pectoris who takes nitroglycerine for chest pain is coping appropriately. The kind of activity precipitating pain and ways to modify this activity might also be investigated by the nurse and client. All opportunities for mutual goal setting should be examined. The nurse who considers the client's chief complaint as important as the client does and is willing to assess and treat that complaint establishes a communication base from which to develop a workable care plan.

The client's perception of the current illness, that is, the meaning it has for him or her, is a very significant determinant of ability to handle this stress. If in the client's view, *cancer* means death, any effort to restore this client to health or to try to maximize wellness during illness will meet with resistance.

In addition, the client's self-image and functional ability can be constructed from questions about the current level and limitations of activity:

1   What is your typical daily activity pattern?
2   Do you need any assistance with these activities?
3   Do you feel you are stable, are improved, or have a decreased tolerance for activity since your last visit?
4   How do you feel your current activity level affects your future?
5   Are you experiencing recent stress, and how are you managing it?

Also, knowledge of family members' illnesses and any genetically linked diseases may be important for the nurse's assessment. Infectious diseases such as tuberculosis can be hazardous to family members living within close proximity to each other.

Some diseases, such as cancer and heart disease, have not been genetically linked but seem to have a familial predisposition. Whether due to social factors or to genetic traits, some ethnic groups are more prone to certain diseases. Jews, for example, have a high incidence of diabetes mellitus, and blacks have a high incidence of hypertension.

Clues to management of current illness can be found in a client's reaction and adjustment to previous illness. The usual information obtained in any history examination, including the problem-oriented examination, is necessary: previous illnesses, operations, accidents, and their dates. In addition, answers to the following questions will give insight into the client's self-image, view of the illness, hospitalization, medical care, coping behaviors, and strengths:

1   Have you been ill previously? When?
2   What was wrong?
3   Were you ill enough to be operated on? If so, what kind of operation did you have? When?

    4 Did you have an accident? If so, when? Where were you hospitalized last?

    5 How long did it take you to recover completely? Do you think your recovery was quick, average, or prolonged?

    6 What kinds of activities (activities of daily living, leisure, work) did you engage in while ill and recovering?

    7 How did you cope with the illness?

    8 How did you cope with decreased activity level, reduced mobility, poor vision, or grief?

    9 What person or persons were most helpful to you during your illness?

    10 How do you feel you were treated by hospital staff during your previous hospitalization?

Because most clients are eager to please and do not want to complain for fear they will not receive the care they need, the answer to the last question may not be completely candid. A person who feels vulnerable and powerless may complain very little.

Some highly significant coping behaviors can be seen in the client's understanding and handling of a therapeutic or normal dietary regime, allergy, medications, pain, and disrupted sleep or bowel habits.

Food has more than nutritional significance to everyone. It has symbolic meaning from cultural and religious standpoints. For most people, eating is a social activity. The geriatric client who usually eats alone may feel more like eating if in the company of friends. The following questions will elicit some facts about food intake and some sociocultural meanings for the observant nurse:

    1 What is your typical day's meal and snack pattern?

    2 Where and with whom do you eat your meals?

    3 What are your food preferences? Are they related to any ethnic or religious customs? (By adopting a diet to a client's preferences as much as possible, one is more likely to get the client to follow the plan of dietary treatment.)

    4 Has the doctor prescribed a special therapeutic diet for you? If so, what do you understand about it? Do you adhere to it all the time? Some of the time? Never? If you deviate, why? Is there some way the nurse or dietitian can help you adhere to it? How does the prescribed dietary regime interfere with your preferred and accustomed eating habits?

    5 Are you over- or underweight? Actual weight is a gross indicator of nutritional health.

    6 Who shops for food in your family? How often is food purchased? In what kind of store is the food purchased? What kind of transportation do you use for food purchasing? (The elderly client may be able to shop for food only once a month in the corner store. Small corner stores have limited choices and higher prices.)

    7 Is anyone else in your family on a special diet?

    8 Who in your family cooks the meals?

The client's knowledge of the expected action, route of administration, and side effects of prescribed medications indicates knowledge of the drugs and also of the disease and its treatment. The client who knows about his or her disease and its treatment feels more in control of things and is able to cooperate more fully. On the other hand, the client with limited or fallacious information about medications, illness, or treatment provides the nurse with a teaching opportunity. The same result can be expected with dietary knowledge.

Self-medication can be a positive or negative potential. Taking acetylsalicylic acid for a headache is appropriate, but not when one is also taking anticoagulants. This is another opportunity for client education.

The following questions about medication are important:

1 What medications, both prescribed and nonprescribed, are you taking? What is the dosage? How often do you take them? How long have you been taking them?
2 What were the doctor's directions for taking the medication? Do you modify them? Sometimes? All the time?
3 Do you experience any side effects for example, drowsiness, from these medications? Have the side effects prevented you from taking the medication the way the doctor has prescribed?
4 Do you understand why the medications were prescribed? Do you see any good effect from taking these medications?
5 Do you find it difficult to meet the cost of these medications? Do you have medications delivered?

The purpose of these questions is to try to determine the client's knowledge of the medications and ability and willingness to take them. Moreover, negative potentials can be turned into positive potentials here. A client may be willing to take the medications and understand their importance, but because of extraneous factors such as cost and transportation be unable to obtain them.

Allergy information, of course, is essential knowledge for the client and nurse as well as for all health care personnel directly involved in care. The following questions are pertinent to the care of a client with an allergy:

1 Do you have any food allergies? If so, what? How are your food allergies manifested? What do you do in case of a reaction?
2 Do you have any medication allergies? If so, what? How are your medication allergies manifested? What do you do in case of a reaction?
3 Are you allergic to any environmental factors, such as pollen or animal dander? How do you manifest this allergy? What do you do for it? (The nurse should be aware of any environmental hazards in the hospital and try to minimize them as much as possible.)
4 Do you wear a Medic Alert bracelet? Do you need to wear one?

Of all the areas of illness-related assessment, the most important and most neglected in terms of readily observable coping behavior is pain response. Everyone who has ever experienced pain has been forced to respond in some manner. Clients cope in some way, and all the nurse needs to do is ask them how. Then it is the responsibility of the nurse to support, modify, or augment the client's own responses.

Pain hurts, and because pain hurts, the person focuses his or her entire attention on the pain and its alleviation. This is another example of the person's unitary reaction to stimuli. The meaning of pain in its physical, cognitive, and affective dimensions significantly determines a person's ability to cope. In the physical dimension, the area affected and the intensity of the pain are proportional to the level of tolerance. A mild headache, for instance, is more easily tolerated than the severe toe pain of gout. The cognitive dimension of pain also determines a client's ability to cope. The client who sees pain after a cholecystectomy as initially severe but ultimately a transitory inconvenience is much more able to tolerate it than is the client who has the chronic, never-ending, nagging pain of low back injury. The ability to tolerate severe stress, in this situation pain, is time-limited.

The affective dimension of pain tolerance can be seen in the client with gastrectomy for an ulcer and the client with bone cancer pain. Both types of pain are severe, but the client with gastrectomy knows the pain is temporary and will diminish, while the cancer client can look forward only to gradual deterioration of the body and sometimes increased pain.

The meaning of pain to a client and the nurse's understanding of that specific meaning will aid in compassionate care. A client who, for example, may think it is shameful to suffer from pain and to be helplessly sick must be understood. The client who thinks that pain is to be endured in stoic silence and who will not take a narcotic for fear of becoming addicted must also be understood. These people will be humiliated if they (1) are in pain so severe they are forced to complain or (2) must ask for a narcotic. Just telling the client it is not shameful to experience pain or take a narcotic for that pain will not eradicate a lifetime of these deep set values. No matter how illogical the client's feelings may seem, they are genuine and the compassionate nurse needs to adapt to them.

During hospitalization, a nurse typically responds to a client's pain cognitively, that is, by administering medication. The nurse does not try to get feedback from the client about what kind of discomfort is experienced. Pain is often the mask of loneliness and fright for many clients. Results of an experimental study by Tarask et al. showed that only 31 percent of clients requesting pain medication really needed it. The remaining 69 percent, although they initially requested pain medication, really had other discomforts more readily alleviated by, for instance, a bedpan, a backrub, or just talking.*

Moreover, nurses in hospitals do not allow clients to use personal coping mechanisms they used at home. Some clients in pain want to pray, pace, moan, or rock. By learning clients' own coping behaviors and allowing them to use

*M. Tarask et al., "An Experimental Test for the Importance of Communication Skills in Effective Nursing," in Skipper, J., and Leonard, R. (eds.), *Social Interaction and Patient Care*, Philadelphia, J. B. Lippincott Co., 1965, p. 112.

them, nurses permit the clients to feel more in control of themselves and their environment, reduce anxiety, and maybe even reduce the subjective feeling of pain: it does not hurt as much.

The following questions provide a glimpse of the client's own pain experience:

1 Do you have pain now? If so, where is it? Describe the pain sensation. Are you taking pain medication? When was your last dose? Do you have any side effects now? Is the medication relieving your pain now?

2 What kind of physical pain have you experienced in the past? What precipitated it? Have you learned to avoid it or to diminish its occurrence or severity? If not, what do you do for the pain?

3 What kind of and how much pain medication do you use? How often do you use it? Do you take the pain medication when in severe pain or moderate pain? How long does it take for the medication to begin working? How long does the therapeutic effect take to wear off? What side effects do you experience?

4 Besides taking medication when you have pain, do you do anything else to augment or enhance the effect of the medication? Do you sometimes omit the pain medication and do something else for the pain, such as taking a hot bath?

Sleep habits are another easily identifiable area of coping. The client who has no problem sleeping at home may be insomniac in the hospital. The routine in the hospital provides basically one way of handling insomniacs: a sleeping pill at 10 P.M. The client who is occasionally or frequently insomniac at home probably has some way of overcoming this problem, for example, a glass of wine, a hot bath, or a cup of tea. The answers to the following questions will help the nurse to understand a client's usual way of handling insomnia at home:

1 What are your normal sleep patterns?

2 How many hours do you sleep at night?

3 Do you ever have trouble getting to sleep at night? What circumstances prevent you from getting to sleep?

4 Do you take sleeping pills? If so, what kind? How often?

5 Do you have any side effects from the sleeping pills?

6 Do you take anything else or do anything else to get to sleep? (While in the hospital, providing some of the same methods of getting to sleep employed at home will help the client maintain a sense of normalcy.)

Social Profile

Most history examinations include information about occupation, age, sex, marital status, amount of alcohol ingested, and smoking habits. However, no information is sought about how the client usually manages life. The social profile is an indicator of social functioning, in other words, how the client manages life.

Demographic data provides a beginning picture of a client's background: the shell from which he or she emerges. Knowledge of growth and development at all age levels can assist the nurse to make inferences about the appropriateness of the client's behavior.

Every age implies certain developmental achievements. One can expect certain levels of intellectual, social, and moral development from different age groups. Tasks, role behaviors, and coping abilities change. A 40-year-old client who usually has difficulty dressing displays grossly inappropriate behavior due to either physical or mental handicap. On the other hand, the 40-year-old person who is employed, enjoys leisure time activities, and has meaningful social interactions displays some of the appropriate developmental achievements of his or her age group.

Age also is important in the care of all clients, especially the dying client. The younger the client the greater is the social loss. An elderly client is seen as having lived a full life, and therefore dying is appropriate, but the death of a child or young adult is seen as unnecessary and cruel.

Even in this age of blurring sex role behaviors, a person's sex is significant in terms of expected life-style, illness, and role behaviors. Women, for instance, live longer and have myocardial infarctions at a later age than men.

The client's educational level, especially language development and ability to communicate, not only indicates cognitive ability for future learning and problem solving but also reveals one ingredient of a general feeling of self-esteem and social competence. Along with education, occupation or social class

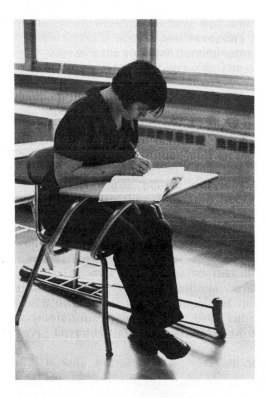

Figure 4-1 In spite of a chronic disabling condition, this person fulfills many developmental tasks, for instance, intellectual mastery.

provides an indication of whether a client has a satisfactory sense of fulfillment of the person's own accomplishments.

As does age, educational level and occupation affect feelings about the dying client. The degree of social loss is proportional to the education and kind of occupation of the dying client. The higher the level of education and the more "professional" or creative the person's background, the greater is the feeling of emotional loss for the survivors, including the staff.

Educational level or occupation notwithstanding, for clients who speak only a foreign language a translator is necessary. Knowledge of frequently used foreign words or other special words in the client's vocabulary is necessary; for instance, even in English many adults and children have special words for urination and defecation.

Another factor that may affect a client's health is occupation. Some people—such as construction workers and miners—have physically dangerous occupations. Other people are employed in positions in which emotional tension is implicit in the job description. How people adjust to the intrinsic emotional and physical dangers of their occupations also provides an indication of their overall health.

The following questions will help the nurse understand the client's job history:

1   Where are you employed? What is your job title? What kind of work does that entail?
2   How do you handle stressful situations on the job?
3   How long have you worked there? Is it a full- or a part-time job? What hours do you work?
4   Do you have more than one job? If so, where is the other job? What do you do? What is your job title? What hours do you work? How long have you worked there?
5   What kind of transportation do you use for work?
6   If you are hospitalized or otherwise unable to work, do sick leave benefits provide adequate temporary income? (If not, a social worker should be notified and alternative plans made for ensuring financial stability.)

If the client is married, similar questions can be asked of the spouse. A spouse's income may be an additional source of support during difficult times.

An occupation has far more than economic value. In some ways, it becomes part of a person's identity, and its loss, for whatever reason, may damage self-esteem and make a person feel worthless. The following questions relate to unemployment:

1   How long have you been out of work?
2   For what reason are you unemployed?
3   Do you consider your unemployment temporary or a prelude to permanent retirement?

The answers to these questions provide more clues to the client's strengths and coping abilities in the face of one kind of adversity, unemployment.

Marital status indicates a level of acceptance of societal norms, but also enables one to make inferences about the acceptance of developmental tasks. Rapoport discusses marriage tasks at length. The pertinent article is listed in this chapter's reading list. The duration of a marriage and the existence of any previous marriages may be an indicator of stability. On another level, friendships and their duration may also be indicators of stability and the potential for closeness or intimacy.

Family interaction can provide essential emotional satisfaction and support or can be very emotionally painful and destructive. Many clients can weather the most severe stresses if they have emotional support at home, but an unstable home life can be the background stress that makes a relatively minor hospitalization very traumatic. The number of family members, their ages, their sexes, and their health are important, along with the kind of home and its general ecological conditions.

The following questions will help clarify some of the family interaction patterns:

1 Are you the breadwinner in the family?
2 Who makes most of the decisions in the household?
3 What kinds of stress do you experience at home?
4 How do you handle these stresses?
5 How are the children included while the ill member is being cared for?
6 Are any other family members ill or in need of care at home?
7 Who takes care of the sick member of the family most of the time?

In addition to family, friends can also provide a sense of interpersonal security and self-esteem. For the single adult in particular, the quality of friendships can be a crucial determinant of the ability or inability to interact meaningfully with others. The following questions help elicit this kind of information:

1 Do you have any close friends?
2 Are you able to express feelings with them?
3 What kinds of things do you do together?
4 Describe your relationship with coworkers.
5 What kinds of social situations do you enjoy?

The nurse needs to ask the client other specific questions relating to support systems. The following questions will elicit information about the support systems:

1 In stressful times to whom do you turn for help? What kinds of help do you receive?
2 What other people or activities make you feel better?

Social and leisure activities indicate a client's interests outside himself or herself and may also indicate acceptance of responsibility for others through participation in organizations. Moreover, social and leisure activities and organizations and groups can be effective support systems. The answers to the following questions will provide information in this regard:

1   What kind of leisure and social activities do you enjoy?
2   Do you belong to any organizations or groups? What significance do they have for you?

Understanding of the spiritual needs of a client can immeasurably enhance the effect of nursing care. Some clients turn to religion for comfort, especially during stressful situations. The client's denomination and the degree to which the religion's ritual and customs are practiced are important information to obtain. Some religions free the ill and handicapped from otherwise required rituals. The following questions may generate more information about support systems:

1   Do you profess to believe in any religion?
2   How does it relate to your daily life?
3   Is your religion a source of strength in times of stress?

The answers to general questions can yield information about overall strengths, self-worth, feelings, and motivations:

1   What are your assets or strengths?
2   What do you like about yourself?
3   What do you do well?
4   Of what are you most proud?
5   What kinds of things interest or motivate you?
6   Are you willing to take risks or chances with the possibility that your life may be improved?
7   How do you think things can be different for you?
8   What are you feeling right now?
9   When you feel angry or sad what do you do?
10 Tell me about a happy and a sad time in your life.

The activities of daily living are also indicators of effective coping behaviors. The person living a very rushed life may need to slow down and look at the reasons why he or she keeps so busy. Alcohol ingestion and smoking may be excessive and therefore self-destructive. The following questions can provide information about life-style satisfaction:

1   Tell me about your daily activities.
2   What in your daily life provides satisfaction?

The nursing assessment culminates in a general summary statement that becomes the nursing diagnosis and includes both the client's and the nurse's view of the client's situation, including ability to cope, impact of the illness on life-style, and identification of major stresses. In relation to strengths the nursing diagnosis should include the ways the client copes with specific problems currently and how this has been done in the past. This extensive nursing history requires much time and developed communication skills. Realistically, a nurse cannot complete it in one interview. Repeated encounters and conversations are needed to add to the picture of the client. Careful recording of observations of and remarks by the client are a necessary part of a complete history and physical.

The strength-oriented nursing record is a preliminary effort to identify some strengths or positive potentials of clients. Olebaum also attempts to look at wellness instead of illness and calls the 26 letters of the alphabet "hallmarks of adult wellness." Each letter of the alphabet relates to an attribute of wellness. For instance, A relates to activities of daily living and O relates to efficient use of oxygen. When coping abilities become more clearly defined, the strength-oriented nursing record will be more specific.

SUMMARY

This chapter has applied the well model to the nursing process. The well model takes the nursing process a step further in that it not only solves problems, but more specifically, it also focuses on the positive aspects of the client. Key concepts in both the well model and the nursing process are integration of the whole person, mutual goal setting, and rights and responsibilities of the client. Whereas the physical problems are more intensified in an episodic setting, these concepts should be equally useful in a distributive setting.

The problem-oriented record has some real value, but its limitations lie in its focus on the sick model: the neglect of clients' strengths, the absence of advocacy, and its semantic misunderstanding of what a problem is (see Bonkowsky).

The four steps of the nursing process are assessing, planning, implementing, and evaluating. Areas that are explored in determining clients' strengths include systems review, illness-related history, and social profile. All the usual methods of data gathering are used. The theoretical framework for the strength-oriented nursing Record includes (1) stress is a part of living, (2) prevailing coping patterns are the result of previous life experiences, (3) the existence and nature of a crisis depend upon a person's relative coping abilities, and (4) stress, when intensified, precipitates more primitive coping responses.

QUESTIONS FOR REFLECTION AND DISCUSSION

4-1 Choose a client. Read his or her history, physical examination, and nursing assessment. Try to identify the client's strengths from this information. Now interview the client using the strength-oriented nursing record. Identify the client's strengths, especially ways of coping with problems, and nursing measures to enhance or support the already present abilities.

4-2 Choose a second client with the same or a similar diagnosis. Follow the same direction as in item 1. Compare and contrast the clients in all areas.

4-3 How does the hospital as an institution enhance or prevent the client from adequately coping with stress? Defend your view.

4-4 Identify coping patterns in yourself.

BIBLIOGRAPHY

Abrams, K. S., Neville, R., and Becker, M. C.: "Problem-Oriented Recording of Psychosocial Problems," *Arcives of Physical Medicine and Rehabilitation*, **54**:316–319, July 1973.

Aradine, C., and Guthneck, M.: "The Problem-Oriented Record in Family Health Service," *American Journal of Nursing*, **74**(6): 1108–1112, June 1974.

Bircher, A.: "On the Development and Classification of Diagnoses," *Nursing Forum*, **14**(1): 10–29, 1975.

Bonkowsky, M.: "Adapting the POMR to Community Child Health Care," *Nursing Outlook*, **20**:515–518, August 1972.

Bower, F.: *The Process of Planning Nursing Care, A Theoretical Model*, St. Louis, C. V. Mosby Co., 1972.

Bruner, J.: *Toward a Theory of Instruction*, Cambridge, Mass., The Belknap Press of Harvard University Press, 1966.

Carlson, S.: "A Practical Approach to the Nursing Process," *American Journal of Nursing*, **72**(9):1589–1591, September 1972.

Erikson, E.: *Childhood and Society*, 2d ed., New York, W. W. Norton Co., 1963.

Glaser, B., and Strauss, A.: "The Social Loss of Dying Patients," *American Journal of Nursing*, **64**(6):119–121, June 1964.

Janis, I.: *Psychological Stress*, New York, John Wiley and Sons, 1958.

Judge, R., and Ziudema, G. (eds.): *Physical Diagnosis: A Physiologic Approach to the Clinical Examination*, Boston, Little, Brown and Co., 1963.

Kübler-Ross, E.: *On Death and Dying*, New York, Macmillan Co., 1969.

Lazarus, R.: *Psychological Stress and the Coping Process*, New York, McGraw-Hill Book Co., 1966.

Lindemann, E.: "Symptomatology and Management of Acute Grief," *American Journal of Psychiatry*, **101**:141–148, September 1944.

Little, D., and Carnevali, D.: *Nursing Care Planning*, 2d ed., Philadelphia, J. B. Lippincott Co., 1976.

MacBryde, C., and Blacklow, R. eds., *Signs and Symptoms, Applied Pathologic Physiology and Clinical Interpretation*, Philadelphia, J. B. Lippincott Co., 1970.

Marriner, A.: *The Nursing Process, A Scientific Approach to Nursing Care*, St. Louis, C. V. Mosby Co., 1975.

Martin, N., et al.: "Nurses Who Nurse," *American Journal of Nursing*, **73**(8):1383–1385, August 1973.

Mauksch, I., and David, M.: "Prescription for Survival," *American Journal of Nursing*, **72**(12):2189–2193, December 1972.

Murray, R., and Zentner, J.: *Nursing Assessment and Health Promotion through the Life Span*, Englewood Cliffs, N.J., Prentice-Hall, 1975.

Olebaum, C.: "Hallmarks of Adult Wellness," *American Journal of Nursing*, 74(9):1623–1625, September 1974.

Phillips, L.: *Human Adaptation and Its Failures*, New York, Academic Press, 1968.

Prior, J., and Silberstein, J.: *Physical Diagnosis*, St. Louis, C. V. Mosby Co., 1969.

Rapoport, R.: "Normal Crisis, Family Structure, and Mental Health," in Parad, H. (ed.), *Crisis Intervention*, New York, Family Service Association of America, 1965, pp. 75–87.

Schaefer, J.: "The Interrelatedness of Decision-Making and the Nursing Process," *American Journal of Nursing*, 74(10):1852–1855, October 1974.

Schell, P., and Campbell, A.: "POMR—Not Just Another Way to Chart," *Nursing Outlook*, 20:510–514, August 1972.

Snyder, J. C., and Wilson, M. F.: "Elements of a Psychological Assessment," *American Journal of Nursing*, 77(2):235–239, February 1977.

Tarask, J., et al.: "An Experimental Test for the Importance of Communication Skills for Effective Nursing," in Skipper, J., and Leonard, R. (eds.), *Social Interaction and Patient Care*, Philadelphia, J. B. Lippincott Co., 1965.

Weed, L.: *Medical Records, Medical Education, and Patient Care; the Problem-Oriented Record as a Basic Tool*, Cleveland, Ohio, The Press of Case Western Reserve University, 1970.

Yura, H., and Walsh, M.: *The Nursing Process, Assessing, Planning, Implementing, Evaluating*, 2d ed., New York, Appleton-Century-Crofts, 1973.

Chapter 5

The Well Model Applied to the Dying Client

In this chapter the well model is made relevant to the care of the dying, especially in relation to the rights of the terminally ill. The remainder of the chapter explores the broad conceptual areas pertinent to the dying process: grief and anticipatory grief, body image, and pain. Fears of the dying are included when related to broad conceptual areas.

THE DYING PROCESS AND THE WELL MODEL

Just as childbirth and growth are normal processes, so, too, are deterioration and death part of the normal cycle of events in every life. Even though dying may follow illness, the well model is still an appropriate way to view the end of a person's life.

Although parts of the body die at different times, the fact remains that the whole body reacts to this process. The concept of wholeness is essential to understanding of both the well model and the dying process. An analogy is helpful: When small portion of the heart muscle dies from an infarction, collateral circulation modifies the coronary circulation to maintain the heart's integrity; to do this adequately the whole body must be at rest for a prolonged period of time. Also, the dying client has many changes to make in life-style.

All the changes must be looked at integrally, as mutually complementary and not mutually exclusive. Everything the client does after the first hard realization of impending death is an effort to maintain equilibrium and control until death.

The dying person's reactions can be viewed in terms of positive and negative potentials, in other words, by the quality of support systems. Maintaining economic stability during a chronic illness, for instance, may help minimize the fear of dependency. On the other hand, an unstable family life may add to the client's feelings of loneliness. People cope with life's exigencies by using their genetic or physical abilities and their psychological development, that is, intellectual processes, social development, and moral development. Intellectual processes are the cognitive abilities to apply concrete and abstract ideas to the real world using inductive and deductive reasoning. Social development concerns a person's relationships with others. Moral development is "the degree to which the person is psychologically capable of accepting reciprocal responsibilities with others."*

RIGHTS OF THE TERMINALLY ILL

Even more than nonterminal clients, clients facing death may be physically too weak or emotionally too upset to assert their rights. The advocate needs to know these rights and provide clients with the opportunity to remain in control of themselves and their environment while dying.

Annas has proposed the most comprehensive and most specific Bill of Rights. He has adapted it to the needs of the terminally ill. He implores physicians and nurses to provide the opportunity for clients to maintain their dignity while dying.

1 *Right to know the truth* The argument surrounding disclosure of diagnosis to a terminal client is still the subject of heated debate among physicians, nurses, and even laypersons. It is interesting to note that the diagnosis is the first thing the physician tells the nonterminal patient.

When a client is labeled "terminally ill," the right to know the truth about the prognosis is often denied. Whether the nondisclosure is in the form of an actual lie, a carefully worded half-truth, or a complete omission and disregard of the client's queries (for instance, "You have nothing to worry about"), it meets the physician's and not the client's needs. The rationales for not telling the truth vary. Some examples are, "He does not really want to know," "We ought to spare him the anguish," "She cannot take it," "She knows anyway," or "We cannot let him give up hope." This nondisclosure sets the stage for denial of the client's rights. In essence, it is the client, not the doctor, who should decide whether he or she wants to know the truth.

2 *Right to confidentiality and privacy* The physician who will not tell a client his or her fate will probably tell a family member. This is a violation of professional confidence. Furthermore, many people, for medical information

*L. Phillips, *Human Adaptation and Its Failure*, New York, Academic Press, 1968, p. 4.

or morbid curiosity, may want to examine the client, especially in a teaching hospital. Of course, learning experiences are not in themselves destructive, but the client who is not given a choice becomes less than a person—just a diagnosis.

Privacy and confidentiality are again violated when discussions in the corridor can be overheard by anyone passing by. Charts can be read by anyone walking into the nurse's station, yet in some states it is difficult if not impossible for clients to see their own charts. Clients are also not allowed to refuse access to their rooms to anyone who wants to chat or just look. Bodily privacy is relinquished and invaded.

3 *Right to consent to treatment*   The physician and nurse need to know that they have done everything for dying clients. The clients, however, need to know that they can refuse that next chemotherapy treatment even if it might give them an outside chance to stay their death.

How often are clients asked if they want to be resuscitated?

> At a minimum the patient should be informed as to what the procedure is and be given the option of directing his doctor to write "no code" on his chart and order card . . . fulfills the patient's right to consent to treatment, and eliminates the covertly penciled "no code" notations erased after the patient has died . . . intensifies public distrust of the medical profession.*

Clients may lose their personhood to the point where they become experiments. They are usually not aware that specimens from their bodies may be used in a future research study. The National Institutes of Health have established guidelines for protecting the rights of human subjects in experiments. These guidelines are not law, but are a matter of ethics and an important step in protecting clients' rights. The new informed-consent laws, in addition, make the physician more accountable to the client. "It is now legally established that a physician can be held liable in an action at law if the patient's consent to treatment has not been an informed consent."† The quality of informed consent is an important issue now being argued. How detailed must a description of a treatment, diagnosis, and prognosis be? In terms of terminal illness the question becomes even more complex: If the doctor does not inform the client that the condition is terminal, can any consent to treatment be considered informed?

4 *Right to choose a place to die*   Over 80 percent of all deaths in the United States occur in hospitals and nursing homes. They have become the socially and medically acceptable places to die. Nursing homes can become dumping grounds for the old when the burden of care becomes too great or too bothersome for the family.

Because of availability of modern equipment and skilled personnel, the terminally ill are usually sent to hospitals. However, it is not necessarily true that a lot of intricate expensive equipment or special training is necessary for

---

*G. Annas, "Rights of the Terminally Ill Patient," *Journal of Nursing Administration*, **42**:42, March-April 1974.
†Ibid.

their care. Nurses can teach family members or paramedical personnel the skills needed for comfort care.

Economics also plays a part in reducing the dying client's choices in relation to a place to die. Hospitalization insurance plans cover hospitalization but sometimes exclude nursing homes and paramedical personnel in the home.

5 *Right to choose the time of death* The change in the legal definition of death, from cardiac to cerebral cessation of function, is an issue that legislatures physicians, and the public must examine.

In 1976 the California Legislature passed the Natural Death Act, giving individuals the legal right to choose to avoid the use of extraordinary measures prolonging life. It is a modification of the Living Will proposed by the Euthanasia Educational Council.

Increasing numbers of people are expressing a wish to choose the manner and time of death. The Euthanasia Educational Council has developed the Living Will (Figure 5-1) as one way in which to do this. When signed, it requests the omission of extraordinary measures to prolong life. This document, in

Figure 5-1 The Living Will.

TO MY FAMILY, MY PHYSICIAN, MY LAWYER, MY CLERGYMAN
TO ANY MEDICAL FACILITY IN WHOSE CARE I HAPPEN TO BE
TO ANY INDIVIDUAL WHO MAY BECOME RESPONSIBLE FOR MY HEALTH, WELFARE OR AFFAIRS

Death is as much a reality as birth, growth, maturity and old age—it is the one certainty of life. If the time comes when I, _____ can no longer take part in decisions for my own future, let this statement stand as an expression of my wishes, while I am still of sound mind.

If the situation should arise in which there is no reasonable expectation of my recovery from physical or mental disability, I request that I be allowed to die and not be kept alive by artificial means or "heroic measures". I do not fear death itself as much as the indignities of deterioration, dependence and hopeless pain. I, therefore, ask that medication be mercifully administered to me to alleviate suffering even though this may hasten the moment of death.

This request is made after careful consideration. I hope you who care for me will feel morally bound to follow its mandate. I recognize that this appears to place a heavy responsibility upon you, but it is with the intention of relieving you of such responsibility and of placing it upon myself in accordance with my strong convictions, that this statement is made.

Signed _____

Date _____

Witness _____

Witness _____

Copies of this request have been given to _____

_____

_____

_____

s a philosophical statement of a commitment to choose the time and
of dying. It is written in vague terms, leaving open to interpretation
such as "heroic measures" and "reasonable expectation." Since the
Living Will is not a legal document, in most states the physician is not bound
by law to honor the client's wishes. Even with its shortcomings, however,
knowledge of a previously signed Living Will may cause a physician to think
twice before initiating life-prolonging measures:

> In general . . . it is the legal right of every mentally competent adult without de-
> pendent children to refuse life-sustaining treatment. Of course, this right is absolute
> while this adult is at home or being treated in an outpatient program (such as kidney
> dialysis). When the patient enters the hospital, this right is necessarily circum-
> scribed, as the hospital staff has a duty to treat·him according to professional
> standards, and he cannot demand mistreatment or demand that his life be affirm-
> atively ended . . .the only way a hospital patient may be able to avoid heroics is
> to demand discharge and go home.*

6 *Right to determine the disposition of his or her body* The family customarily signs an autopsy permit after death. In so doing, the client's predeath
wishes may or may not be taken into account. Here is an example of a client
exerting his legitimate rights: When facing high-risk surgery he insisted upon
signing his own autopsy permit. This was an unusual occurrence, and it somewhat unnerved the staff. However, he was well within his rights.

The Uniform Anatomical Gift Act, now law in all 50 states, compels both
physician and family to heed the client's predeath wishes regarding organ do-
nation and transplant. Clients who want their organs donated or transplanted
carry a card with them (Figure 5-2). As of July 1, 1976, fourteen states permit
a person when renewing a driver's license to have stated on the license that
he or she is an organ donor, in the event of a fatal accident. In actual practice,
though, the wishes of an objecting family will usually prevail.

DYING-RELATED CONCEPTS

A discussion of crisis, grief and loss, body image, and pain is essential to
understanding of the dying client's rights. Together these are the major concepts
with which the client's nurse must work if care of the dying is to be understood.
Within this framework the fears of the dying will be examined.

Crisis

The literal meanings of the word *crisis* provide a basis from which to develop
an understanding of the dying client. In medicine, for example, a crisis is a
highly unstable condition: that change in a disease that indicates whether the
result is to be recovery or death. Therefore, the potential threat of disintegration
and death is an essential property of crisis. On the other hand, as Rapoport
emphasizes, a crisis is *not* an illness and *is* an opportunity for growth. Inter-

*Ibid., p. 43.

Figure 5-2 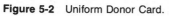 Uniform Donor Card.

UNIFORM DONOR CARD

OF _____
                        Print or type name of donor

In the hope that I may help others, I hereby make this anatomical gift, if medically acceptable, to take effect upon my death. The words and marks below indicate my desires.

I give: (a) —— any needed organs or parts

           (b) —— only the following organs or parts

_____
                        Specify the organ(s) or part(s)

for the purposes of transplantation, therapy, medical research or education;

           (c) —— my body for anatomical study if needed.

Limitations or
special wishes, if any: _____

Signed by the donor and the following two witnesses in the presence of each other:

_____   _____
        Signature of Donor   Date of Birth of Donor

_____   _____
        Date Signed   City & State

_____   _____
          Witness   Witness

This is a legal document under the Uniform Anatomical Gift Act or similar laws.

estingly, "in Chinese, the character that means crisis is made up of two characters, one meaning danger, and the other, opportunity."* (See Figure 5-3.)

Caplan and Lindemann feel that a crisis is the state of the individual's
reacting to a hazardous event. This hazardous situation takes the form of a
threat, loss, or challenge:

> The threat may be to fundamental, instinctual needs or to the person's sense of
> integrity. The loss may be actual or may be experienced as a state of acute dep
> rivation. For each of these states there is a major characteristic mode in which the
> ego tends to respond. A threat to need and integrity is met with anxiety. Loss or
> deprivation is met with depression. If the problem is viewed as a challenge, it is
> more likely to be met with a mobilization of energy and purposive problem-solving
> activities. . . . The crisis with its mobilization of energy operates as a second chance
> in correcting earlier faulty problem-solving.†

This hazardous event requires coping abilities that may not have been used
in the past. With no previous experience of dying, the client may not have
adequate coping resources without external intervention.

Every individual, however, has developed some patterns of coping with
stress, and these are essential to maintainence of equilibrium:

> Resulting tension-reducing mechanisms, both overt and covert, may be ones of
> aggression, withdrawal, regression, repression . . . the choice being based upon
> effective, learned, tension-reducing responses to other situations in the past.‡

Another characteristic of a crisis is the inadequacy of customary problem-
solving mechanisms in meeting the needs of the current situation. In well model
terms, a crisis is an opportunity to turn negative potentials into positive, growth-
promoting potentials.

Historically, crisis intervention began with the emergence of community
psychiatry, and gradually hospitals saw value in the techniques. A person can
experience a crisis in or out of the hospital. A crisis can occur in the delivery
room, with a stillbirth; in the emergency room, after an automobile accident;
during cardiac arrest; or when a loved one is dying after a protracted illness
while at home or institutionalized. Traditional methods of crisis intervention
may need to be modified for the hospital. Use of crisis intervention in the
acutely dying setting and in the chronically dying setting will be discussed in
the following chapters.

*I. Taves, *Love Must Not Be Wasted; When Sorrow Comes Take It Gently by the Hand*,
New York, Thomas Y. Crowell Co., 1974, p. 175.

†L. Rapoport, "The State of Crisis: Some Theoretical Considerations," in Parad, H. (ed.),
Crisis Intervention, Selected Readings, New York, Family Service Association of America, 1965,
p. 25.

‡D. Aguilera, "Crisis: Death and Dying," in *ANA Clinical Sessions*, New York, Appleton-
Century-Crofts, 1968, p. 276.

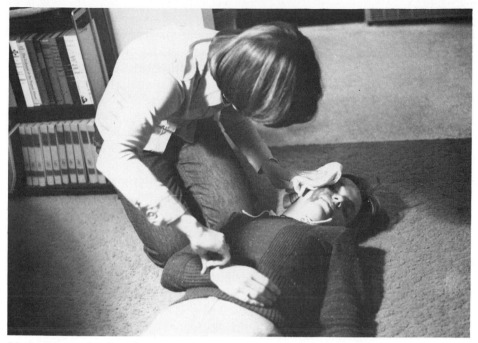

(a) A crisis may be viewed as a challenge. . .

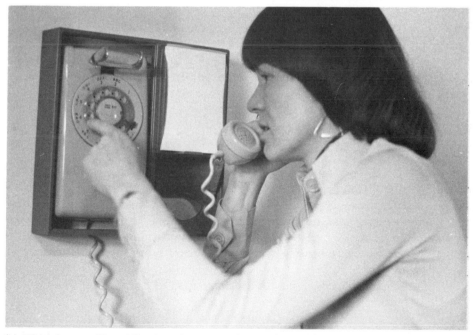

(b) Which is met with mobilization of energy and purposive problem-solving activity

Figure 5-3   Dynamics of crisis.

Dying can be viewed from both a situational and a maturational perspective. The situational perspective is the illness, long or short, superimposed on the normal maturational process. At certain times, during periods of definable change, such as adolescence, middle age, or senility, the person is especially vulnerable. An illness adds to the stress of maturational changes (Erickson calls these changes *developmental* or *normative crises*), leading to an increasingly unstable and potentially disorganizing effect on the client, family, and staff. Erikson's view of the last stage of man as appropriate for dealing with death is incomplete. It is also a normal developmental task of adolescence and all other ages to face death in self and others. Possibly that progressive understanding of the meaning of death culminates in the elderly's person's meeting death with equanimity.

Clients cope in a manner in which they have handled their previous life experiences. Any illness can profoundly affect normal, maturational task performance. Sometimes return to the preillness state is possible, as, for example, after a fractured leg. At other times return to the preillness state is not possible, and adjustment to the chronicity of the illness is a major task. Goals may have to be severely modified or abandoned altogether in the adjustment to a life-shortening chronic illness.

The nurse need not be a psychotherapist to use crisis theory and crisis-intervention techniques in the care of the dying client. The *generic method* of crisis intervention has been successfully used by other professionals. It involves directly encouraging adaptive behavior, generally supporting, manipulating the environment, and preparing the client for future stresses. It "focuses on the characteristics of the particular kind of crisis rather than on the psychodynamics of the individual in crisis."*

The other method of crisis intervention, *individual*, emphasizes professional assessment of interpersonal and intraphysic processes of the client. Both types of intervention seek to improve the precrisis emotional state and coping abilities. Crisis intervention is an opportunity for learning for both the client and the intervenor. Dying is one of the special times when help is needed because equilibrium is severely threatened.

In the schematic diagram in Chapter 3, crisis unfreezes the current situation and a period of instability ensues. The need to change is identified in the desire to resolve the crisis and return to a period of equilibrium or stability. Specific goals must be agreed upon by the person in crisis and the nurse or other team member. The client's strength or positive potentials must be supported. The effect of the negative potentials can be minimized by proper assessment and intervention.

The well model nursing process is analogous to the steps in crisis intervention. The first step, assessment, attempts to define the problem and elicit coping mechanisms and other valuable resources. The second and third steps,

*D. Aguilera and J. Messick, *Crisis Intervention, Theory and Methodology*, 2d ed., St. Louis, C. V. Mosby Co., 1974, p. 17.

planning and intervention, set forth and execute care necessary to return the client to the state of equilibrium. The plan may include discussion, medication, environmental manipulation, or specific direction. The final step is evaluation and anticipatory planning. How well has the situation been resolved? How can what the client has learned from this situation help in subsequent threatening situations?

> Much of the effectiveness of crisis intervention lies in the humanity of the intervenor and his positive attitude toward the strengths of the person in crisis. Actual words are of relatively little significance. Crisis therapy is not depth therapy, but dealing supportively with here and now issues. This takes skill and a fund of knowledge, but not an extensive theoretical and experiential background in psychiatry or psychiatric nursing. Any nurse with warm feelings toward patients, ability to express her belief in another human, and sufficient interest to learn the simple steps can offer effective crisis intervention.*

Partial Deaths, Anticipatory Grief, and Grief

Loss is involved in partial deaths, anticipatory grief, and grief and mourning. Every person must adjust to a series of, in Shneidman's term, *partial deaths* before experiencing the final loss of self in death. These partial deaths cannot be considered pathological, but occur in the normal course of a lifetime. Successful mastery of a lifetime of partial deaths may aid in mastery of the final dying process.

Developmentally, a universal loss for the child is the relinquishing, not without some trauma, of bottle or breast for cup or glass. Social or psychological losses affect the relationship of self to the outside world. For the adolescent, the body-image change that comes with physical maturation includes changes in social roles and tasks. The adolescent experiences loss of previous body image and appearance. For the adult, resolution of the experience of a partial loss, for instance, the loss of a job or a spouse, requires the birth of a slightly different identity. Just as parturition is more difficult for some women than others, so these partial deaths are more difficult for some people than for others. Obviously, the meaning a loss has for a person greatly affects its impact and eventual resolution. These losses can occur in all spheres of living.

Change that occurs with early developmental partial deaths elicits a kind of grieving, and so does change in relation to the dying client. The dying person grieves for accumulated actual and anticipated losses, such as loss of economic independence, loss of health, and loss of loved ones.

At any point a crisis may result through the acute realization of these losses. Nevertheless, grieving begins at the first awareness of loss. *Grief* can

---

*J. Hitchcock, "Crisis Intervention, the Pebble in the Pool," *American Journal of Nursing*, 73(8):1388–1390, August 1973.

be defined as a total response of profound sadness and emptiness for irreversible loss of a loved or valued object. That loved or valued object can be health, a bodily part, the self, self-worth, an occupation, a relationship, or a tangible possession such as a house. Grief takes the form of a patterned desocialization, whereby the survivor "achieves emancipation from the bondage of the deceased, readjustment to the environment in which the deceased is missing and the formation of new relationships."* *Mourning* is generally considered to be the intraphysic processes that are involved in grief and should lead to integration and healthy resolution of the loss. *Bereavement* is the state of mourning after the death of a person.

Anticipatory grief, which has many similarities to actual grief, is the sadness for future anticipated losses. The significant difference between the two concepts is hope and reversibility. As long as the loss does not now exist, one can hope that the inevitable will be delayed. That denial and acceptance of loss existing side by side in the client and the significant people around are the basis of anticipatory grief. Weisman calls this *middle knowledge*. Just as the ambivalence of the love-hate relationship with those close to each person brings conflict, the acceptance/denial of the dying client is a source of intrapsychic discomfort and conflict. This, then, is a capsule view of the grief work of the client who knows he or she has a terminal illness. Anticipatory grief is an essential part of the letting go process of dying. If one isn't told one is dying, the inevitable partial losses are more mystifing.

Many factors affect a person's response to loss. The affective importance or symbolic meaning attached to the loss can intensify or minimize grieving. The death of an acquaintance has a far milder impact than the death of a spouse. Previous experience with loss may be especially important if incompletely resolved. Reawakening very painful memories can leave a person with a lessened feeling of self-control and effectiveness. This is an especially poignant and difficult problem for the health care worker who must repeatedly face death with clients. Nevertheless, ethnic, economic, religious, and cultural patterns provide acceptable models of grieving. A person's pattern of adaptation to life changes and to loss in particular also affects grieving patterns. Some people seem to adapt to change with less disruption and difficulty than others. Age and social value also affect grieving.

Stage Theory   It is customary to break down the dying process into a series of *stages*. *Dying*, then, becomes the unifying concept to which a person is reacting. These stages have value in that they expose the various emotions a person experiences while dying.

On the other hand, there are some problems with stage theory. Stages are convenient ways to pigeonhole and formularize clients' behavior. To pigeonhole or formularize care is to take a theoretical notion and inflexibly apply it to a

---

*E. Lindemann, "Symptomatology and Management of Acute Grief," *American Journal of Psychiatry*, **101**:143, September 1944.

client. Actually the client is fitted to the theory. Kübler-Ross's stage theory of dying fosters formularizing and neglects the individual attributes of the client in favor of identifying the stages. In fairness to Kübler-Ross, she does state that not everyone goes through these stages in sequence and that the time span is flexible. These are the basic stages (see Table 5-1):

1 *Denial* The client cannot believe that the diagnosis is true. A sense of numbness of affect is apparent.

2 *Anger* When conscious realization of the diagnosis occurs, anger may be directed at God, the physician, nurse or family.

3 *Bargaining* The client will ask God to extend life for a specific period of time if the person does some good work.

4 *Depression* Feelings of sadness occur over the reality of the anticipated loss. The person may become less communicative.

5 *Acceptance* This stage is not resignation, but a surrender and lack of feeling.

Staging implies an invariant pattern of emotional and behavioral change in the dying client. However, not enough research has been done to warrant this assumption. More information on individual variations in adaptation and coping would provide a more comprehensive view of the emotions of the dying client. In this heterogenous Western culture, there may be many normal patterns, depending upon the many highly individual circumstances in a person's life. On the surface it appears that even customary mood patterns can be classified and categorized, but this classification results in an oversimplification of the total experience which produces gaps in perception and in understanding actual problems clients exhibit or keep hidden. A theory of emotional changes that provides for individual variability is acceptable. How relevant is staging, for instance, to non-Western cultures? Can staging be duplicated in American Indian or Australian aborigine culture? This has yet to be validated.

Another fallacious assumption about stage theory, derived specifically from Kübler-Ross's work, is that the nurse must identify the stage the client is in

Table 5-1 Stages of Grieving

Engle: Loss	Kübler-Ross: Anticipatory grief of dying	Gullo et al.: Life threat responses (cancer)
1. Shock and disbelief	1. Denial	1. Shock
2. Developing awareness of loss	2. Anger	2. Anger
3. Restitution	3. Bargaining (magical thinking)	3. Grief and anticipatory grief
	4. Depression	4. Bargaining
	5. Acceptance	5. Uncertainty
		6. Renewal and rebuilding
		7. Integration of experience

and herd the client through it. It is not the responsibility of the nurse to help the client over these stages, like a horse going over hurdles. With such an attitude the nurse attempts to retain control over the client. Nor can the nurse expect a client to be open just because the nurse would like his or her client to talk about dying. The nurse must return control to the client and not feel personally and professionally defeated if the person does not want to talk. One cannot assume, also, that a person who is not in an identifiable "stage" is maladapting.

Moreover, staging does not attempt to consider individual personality styles and coping mechanisms. In a very small study that researched responses to life-threatening illness, Gullo et al. found results similar to Kübler-Ross's and also found predominant response styles, or an "enduring mode of response to life-threatening illness."* The examples of predominant response styles are death-accepter, death-submitter, death-denier, death-defier, and death-tran-scender. Each of these styles is an "underlying behavioral theme enduring through the different stages.† In other words, overall personality patterns could be identified throughout all these stages. These patterns become the prevailing learned and now intrinsic coping patterns. It remains for further research to describe whether stage theory is superimposed on personality patterns or vice versa.

There is also a temporal problem with stage theory. The chronically dying person takes months and sometimes years to die in contrast to the acutely dying person, who is dead in a few minutes, hours, days, or weeks. Kübler-Ross's stage theory was formulated from interviews with chronically dying clients. To them time was available for anticipatory grief work. For the acutely dying, time may not be available to work through the stages or they may be worked through very quickly. The problems of the acutely dying client in the critical care setting have not been adequately addressed.

Engle has identified three broad stages of grieving, into which Kübler-Ross's stages of dying and Gullo et al.'s life-threatened stages can be placed (see Table 5-1 for a comparison of the three systems). Moreover, Engle has incorporated parts of Lindemann's classic work on grief and bereavement into the stages. Engle's stages are broad enough to represent responses to loss in general, including bereavement, anticipatory grief, and adaptation to chronic illness and body-image change.

Engle's Stages of Grieving (see Table 5-1)

1 *Shock and disbelief* There is an immediate denial of loss because of overwhelming stress and threat. The range of feeling extends from an immediate "No," "It can't be" to the later numbed feelings and automatic fulfillment of

*S. Gullo et al., "Suggested Stages and Response Styles in Life-Threatening Illness: A Focus on the Cancer Patient," in Schoenberg, B., et. al (eds.), *Anticipatory Grief*, New York, Columbia University Press, 1974, p. 78.
†Ibid., p. 67.

necessary activities. Or the person may sit motionless. During occasional moments when feeling penetrates, despair and anguish may take over. This phase extends from minutes to days and provides a necessary protective mechanism in the face of very painful loss.

2 *Developing awareness of loss* With increasing awareness of loss, physical symptoms such as an empty feeling in the epigastrium or the chest, may result. The reaction may be a combination of sadness, anger, guilt, and crying. A person's cultural background provides socially acceptable behaviors in which grief is manifested.

3 *Restitution—The work of mourning* Culturally prescribed rituals such as the funeral are important supports in mourning and serve symbolic, personal, social, and religious purposes. The mourner feels a painful void, as if a part of himself or herself were lost. Physical symptoms may appear, sometimes resembling those symptoms the deceased experienced prior to death. Preoccupation with thoughts of the dead person is necessary to eventually put into perspective the lost relationship and its positive and negative qualities. After many months thoughts of the deceased become less frequent and the survivor is again able to be comfortable and to enjoy new objects and activities.

Engle is not all-inclusive in his description of acute grief reactions, and therefore it is necessary to look at Lindermann's work. Although he did not specifically stage bereavement, his original classic research on grief identified specific signs and symptoms in bereaved survivors. Of course individual variations exist, but on the whole these signs and symptoms are remarkably uniform. Since Lindemann's work, done in the early forties, grief has often been referred to as an illness. The signs and symptoms of acute grief include sighing respirations, lack of strength and exhaustion, digestive symptoms, a slight sense of unreality, a feeling of increased emotional distance from other people, intense preoccupation with the image of the deceased, feelings of guilt, loss of warmth in relationships with other people, rapid speech, restlessness, and an inability to initiate and maintain meaningful activity. Some bereaved individuals even take on the behavior traits and illness symptoms of the deceased.

Psychiatrists Lindemann and Engle view grief from the psychoanalytic model. Engle also views grief as an illness and equates it with a wound. Viewing grief as an illness, that is, through the sick model, the focus is on the signs and symptoms of the disease and not on the strengths of the mourner who is coping with a profound loss with a moderate-to-severe degree of disequilibrium. Continuing to put grief into perspective, more recent writers have broadened and lengthened what is considered the ''normal'' process of grief and mourning. It is important to understand that there is no generally recognized specific time period for the completion of grief work.

Morbid and pathological mourning must be viewed with the above perspective in mind. The following are some of the most commonly viewed manifestations of morbid or pathological mourning, excerpted from Lindemann: (1) delayed reactions sometimes involving years; (2) distorted reactions: overactivity without a sense of loss, symptom indentification, an actual medical condition such as ulcerative colitis, progressive social isolation, furious hostility against specific persons, schizophrenic symptoms masking hostility, lack of decision-making power and initiative in social interaction, acts that are self-punitive and detrimental to one's own social and economic existence, and agitated depression.

Engle also adds as evidence of unsuccessful grieving the following manifestations: (1) denial of death, that is, acting and speaking as if the person were still alive; (2) denial of the loss or of the affect, for example, failure to cry, but failure to cry in public is not necessarily pathological since most people save their crying for private times [see Figure 5-4]; (3) use of a vicarious object, as in feeling sorry for someone else who is mourning instead of for oneself, or quick replacment of the lost object with someone else; (4) prolonged unresolved grief, sometimes called *chronic grief*, in which the slightest mention of the deceased, even many years later, readily evokes crying. Also, anniversary reactions, that is, the reawakening of unresolved grief precipitated by mutual special occasions, are common but are not always pathological. Too, sometimes the mourner refuses to change any of the deceased's physical environment, such as clothes or home, awaiting the deceased's return.

To assist the pathological mourner, regrief therapy is used. It is a kind of brief psychotherapy that attempts to help the mourner remember the loss and its affect, grow to accept the affect, and put the loss in perspective.

Figure 5-4 Crying is a normal, healthy response to the awareness of loss.

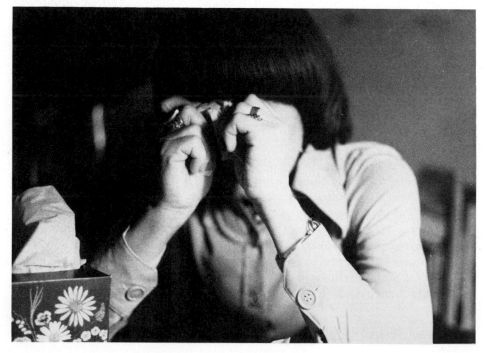

Another theorist, Weisman, views the dying process from a little different perspective. He does not stage dying but places the various fluctuating kinds of denial at different levels. They are as follows:

First-order denial is unequivocal repudiation of the facts of a situation, such as the diagnosis.

Second-order denial occurs when the facts of illness are accepted but the implications are denied, often with rationalizations.

Third-order denial occurs when the diagnostic facts and implications are accepted but eventual death is not. Only the diagnosis is communicated to the significant people in the person's life, to spare them the anguish of death.

To reiterate, if one looks at grief as a series of complex fluctuating emotions or feelings and not as clearly defined stages, it is easier to identify the person experiencing these feelings. The person who is grieving needs understanding and the freedom to experience feelings in whatever order they come. There is no one right way to grieve.

In terms of the well model, the grieving process is an unstable, unfrozen situation. The need for change can be seen in the efforts of the griever to experience the loss and learn to readjust to life with this knowledge. The willingness to talk and the willingness to listen are essential mutual goals. The strengths, or positive potentials, remaining must be supported. The newly bereaved, for instance, should be encouraged to remain in the same home. Negative potentials, such as sudden loss of income when a family breadwinner dies, may be minimized by consultative efforts by the social service department.

Body Image

The concept of body image is helpful in our viewing of the dying client as a totality. Everyone has a body image. It is the totality of one's sense of oneself, including one's physical body, self-concept, and relationships to others. Another way of expressing body image is "intrapersonal experience of the person's feelings and attitudes towards one's body and the way he organizes these experiences."* The inevitable changes in body image that occur during the illness and dying process must be integrated by the person if adaptive and eventually coping efforts are to be made to achieve mastery and continued control over self.

Normal and developmental aspects Body image cannot be understood in terms of normality or abnormality because "differences between what is considered to be a healthy presentation of the body image and its pathological variants are not generally specified or known."†

Beginning with the pleasure and pain experiences of infancy, which em-

*C. Norris, "The Professional Nurse and Body Image," in Carlson, C. (ed.), *Behavioral Concepts and Nursing Intervention*, Philadelphia, J. B. Lippincott Co., 1970, p. 42.
†Ibid.

anate from internal structures and external environmental sources, and progressing to the slowing down that occurs with aging, body image is a total and often unconscious experience. It has also been called the *somatic ego*:

> [The] goals are manipulation, mastery and control of relationships with self, others and environment within a time-space context or rhythm . . . forming newer, more stable systems in the organism. However, under stress older ways of interpretating and functioning in relation to the body image may be revived.*

Not only is body image related to development, but it also is related to the health-sickness continuum. During the nursing assessment the client, in describing illness-related facts combined with social profile, can reveal information about body image, including description of daily patterns and usual coping behaviors in the face of illness. The person, for example, who has had surgery several times in the last few years for gallbladder, bunions, inguinal hernia, and tooth extractions may feel "sickly" and expect complications from the current hospitalization. In contrast, the person who has been paraplegic for 10 years and now enters the hospital for gallbladder surgery may feel "healthy" and expect to have routine surgery and be out of the hospital in 2 weeks. The former client may feel much more threatened than the latter client. The body image of the latter client retains a more positive connotation.

Norris suggests that "the most useful attitude for the nurse to assume is to regard the patient as . . . coping, in however inadequate way . . . to . . . an overwhelming experience."† Labeling the client "disoriented," for example, makes the attempt to identify coping mechanisms more difficult.

When entering the sickness care setting, clients probably view themselves as sick and in need of help. This "sick role" is partly a social creation. The sick person is expected by society to seek help, become dependent, and then become well. Normal tasks are abrogated for a more dependent and in many ways childlike role. Persons who temporarily resist the sick role increase the stress on themselves because they are unable to accept help, and their behavior patterns may make the person sicker.

Both ethnic background and economic status also have an effect on body image. Some cultures value obese women; therefore, being emaciated would make a woman feel abnormal, out of place, and maybe offensive. It would be a threat to body image and its emotional counterpart, self-esteem. Norms of youth, wholeness, and beauty pervade homogenized middle-class culture. Any threat to these values by aging, sickness, surgery, or deformity does violence to a person's body image.

Adaptation to body-image change   There are many variations in the adaptational process of coping with body-image change. Commonly, clients first

*Ibid.
†Ibid., p. 59.

request to see the changed body part, peeking at the changed part or looking at it through a mirror. Next, they verbally test the persons closest to them. The clients are both fascinated and repulsed and need to be reassured of social acceptability. Nurses may be the first people tested. Also, clients can verbally maneuver respondents into giving a positive reply by saying, for example, "The scar will not look as bad later, will it?"

Denial may be necessary when the threat is too great at present to handle. It may surface in disguised forms, such as a feeling of emptiness, a vague feeling of weakness, fatigue, vulnerability, intractable pain, hypochondriasis, nervousness, obsession, or phobias. These symptoms are similar to those experienced while grieving.

Norris summarizes the nature of the threats of any body-image change:

1   Threat of being found inadequate in meeting the changes of normal growth and maturational processes
2   Threat to the cultural values of youth, wholeness, normality, and attractiveness
3   Threat presented by changing patterns of adaptation, and impact of the symbolic meanings of organs affected by the changes, for example, uterus or breasts
4   Threat of "degree to which loss of functional control creates loss of customary control over self, physical environment, time and interpersonal field"*
5   Threat to self from subjective meaning of curative procedure or treatment, for instance, equating of anesthesia with loss of control over one's body
6   Threat to self from possible social rejection

The dying client and body image   Changes in body image in the dying person should be viewed as adaptations to partial and multiple deaths. Some of the fears of the dying imply body-image changes: pain, mutilation, dependency, abandonment, loneliness, and the unknown.

Any visible scar, whether it is on the face or on the abdomen and usually hidden, as well as any amputation or surgical alteration of function can be considered a mutilation. As their physical condition deteriorates, clients become visibly more unattractive. The nurse has a difficult task reassuring them that they are acceptable, worthy, and lovable in the face of a mirror that says "ugly." So they look at themselves, feel revulsion, and cry. They now expect rejection and may actually be rejected by social contacts, possibly even by their families, which only increases the sense of loneliness. Could today be a preview of tomorrow? Does it hold further mutilation, pain, loneliness, and rejection?

As illness progresses, the clients lose strength and functional ability and become increasingly dependent upon others. This loss of control over them-

*Ibid., p. 54.

selves and their world robs the clients of self-esteem. They are now washed, toileted, and fed by others, often strangers.

Because of their loss of energy they cannot actively seek out companionship. Family and friends must be relied upon to take the initiative. They may be financially dependent upon spouse or children because of an inability to work and the drain of medical costs.

The clients' moods may not always be pleasant, and, of course, an unpleasant mood affects the family. Interatction with the clients becomes more difficult. Staff and family feel helpless. They also grieve. As a result, a family visits less frequently. The staff enter the room only when necessary. Increasing isolation leads clients to feel lonely and abandoned. They have lost their loved ones. In contrast to the Freudian idea that fear of death is primary, Aldrich feels that loss of loved ones may be of greater concern to the dying than actual fear of death. During a protracted illness a family can even complete grieving before the client dies. Then the family visits even less, only leaving the client to feel more isolated. Finally the fears of the future loneliness, abandonment, and loss of loved ones are a painful reality.

From a well model perspective, body-image change is a fluid situation. A new body image is emerging as a result of the illness process. A client needs to grieve over the lost body image. The mutual goal is an acceptable (to the client) body image. Positive potentials and strengths can be supported by (1) helping the client to maintain previously successful ways of coping with change (found in the strength-oriented nursing record), (2) encouraging social contacts, especially with the family, and (3) encouraging as much independent activity as possible. Reassurance that a measure of normalcy is possible can be reinforced by a visitor from a voluntary organization who has the same condition. Negative potentials can be minimized by early assessment and intervention. If insomnia, for instance, is a problem, many ways to intervene are possible. The nurse may refer to the strength-oriented nursing record for information on how the client usually copes with insomnia at home, or a backrub or a relaxing conversation may help.

Pain

For the terminal client pain can be a major problem. Moderate to severe pain will immobilize a person so that final days and nights are a nightmarish litany of "Is it time yet?" or "When is my next pain medication due?" Some cancer clients die in pain. But pain is also a factor in angina, in decubitus ulcers from prolonged bedrest, and in arthritis in the elderly. People don't die of pain; they just suffer.

Pain evokes more than primary or cognitive perception. First, pain response requires intact neural pathways. Physiological changes of pain perception, such as increased pulse and blood pressure, are accompanied by behavioral and emotional changes aimed at reducing or diminishing the impact of the pain.

The subjective perception of pain provokes a response that is a little different in each person. Results of research on pain thresholds are mixed; some researchers say that pain thresholds vary from person to person and culture to culture, but others found no significant difference in pain thresholds.

Culture seems to have an effect on pain perception and response. Some cultures permit and provide far more noticeable responses to pain. Jews and Italians, for instance, are more verbal in their response to pain than are Chinese or Anglo-Saxon Americans. This generalization can only foster stereotyping, though. The nurse must look at aspects of pain response other than culture to adequately evaluate the client in pain.

A person in pain attaches powerful symbolic meaning to that pain: either dysfunction, alteration, or loss of a part of the body that used to be healthy and pain-free. The affected organ or part may have functional or sexual significance; therefore, pain in that organ means diminished functional ability or sexual attractiveness. For instance, a painful leg means loss of independence and mobility. If the threat of pain in an existing leg is great, then phantom leg pain is much more of a threat, because the person is aware of the amputation, the total loss, but still feels pain as if the leg were still there. Other examples include postmastectomy pain or pain of a myocardial infarction. Both these kinds of pain have implications for both sexuality and death.

A mastectomy may cause a person to feel sexually less attractive and fear eventual death from metastasis. A myocardial infarction may cause a person to fear immediate death or death from a recurrence of the problem. After a myocardial infarction a person may fear inability to perform sexually or that sexual activity may precipitate another coronary and death.

In Copp's study clients attached many meanings to pain. To some clients, pain had redeeming value in the form of a challenge, or made them appreciate previous good health, or helped them identify with other persons who have suffered. Many clients felt that pain and suffering had strong religious significance. For some, chest pain meant punishment, weakness, loss, an enemy, or helplessness. Persons in pain also experienced a loss of control over themselves.

In addition to understanding cognitive and affective aspects of pain, the nurse must also understand clients' previous experience with pain and their residual feelings about it. Of prime importance in dealing with the current pain situation is the clients' own effort to cope with the pain. Copp discovered several coping styles clients used before and during pain. During the prodormal phase of pain, methods used to reduce pain intensity were strenuous work or play, motionlessness, or repeated recitation of certain words that focused on some other activity. Clients timed medication intake and used physical measures such as application of heat and cold, special breathing exercises, rocking, pacing, and many other activities.

The most common response to actual pain, in Copp's study, was vigilant focusing. She mentions six major types of vigilant focusing. One, some clients counted objects or numbers. Two, some clients used words in various ways, for instance, to plead or intercede, to memorize, or to hypnotically repeat nonsense words. Three, deep thinking included praying; visualizing shadows, shapes, and colors; and imagining such activities as sewing or traveling. Four, the deliberate separation of mind and body was attempted by "quitting the mind," "letting the body drop away," and "helping the body escape." Five, smoking or talking to others were some activities clients used to distract themselves from the pain. Six, other people, such as roommates, were thought to be helpful when one was in pain.

Many methods have been and continue to be used for pain relief. A few examples are acupuncture, biofeedback, electrical stimulation, hypnosis, and surgery. The most commonly used method is the chemical one, that is, pharmacologic agents. Narcotics and nonnarcotic analgesics are the agents most commonly used when the request is specifically for pain medication.

Antianxiety, antidepressant, and psychedelic agents are used to keep the dying client comfortable. Kübler-Ross states that sometimes the amount of medication a client receives is proportional to the amount of discomfort the staff feel. The more uncomfortable the staff feel, the more medication the client receives. This keeps the staff from confronting their own feelings.

Even with all the modalities used, adequate pain relief continues to be a problem for clients in American hospitals. The essential need for pain relief more often than not is left unmet because physicians write medication orders with very little flexibility. The client must wait the required 3 or 4 hours for the next dose even if the therapeutic effect has disappeared. Adequate pain relief is a problem with many facets, not the least of which is fear of addiction.

In contrast, there is one hospital in which the terminally ill receive pain relief without even asking. Saint Christopher's Hospice in London provides a sliding dosage scale of analgesics on a routine basis at the times the clients think they need the medication most, for instance, at mealtime and bedtime. They do not have to wait until the pain is unbearable. Nurses use their judgment in increasing or decreasing dosage as needed. A variety of agents are used, including heroin, alcohol, and, of course, narcotic analgesics.

Recent experiments in terminal care have developed previously maverick ideas into viable projects. With governmental permission and under strict control, a research team in Catonsville, Maryland, administered lysergic acid diethylamide (LSD) to persons with cancer. The experiences under the influence of LSD helped clients, when returning to reality, come to terms with their own deaths. On the whole, more imaginative efforts in addition to those at St. Christopher's Hospice and at Catonsville need to be made before we can say that nurses' ministrations are comfort-producing and anguish-allaying. The client in pain cannot complete many other necessary tasks before dying, since without adequate pain relief a person can focus on little else.

Nurses can begin by understanding clients' pain, by allowing them to use their coping mechanisms, and by teaching alternative coping mechanisms. With practice, they can provide a listening ear even though the words are uncomfortable to hear. Nurses can augment clients' coping mechanisms with medications, when needed, and backrubs. Moreover, if clients in pain do not want to be left alone, nurses should remain with them. Active participation by clients in their care is the keystone of the well model. However, they cannot participate actively if overcome with pain.

In terms of the well model, pain is a negative potential. The body's reaction to pain is total, and therefore persistent severe pain can interfere significantly with enjoyment of daily activities. To prevent disequilibrium and minimize the effects of pain, nurses can allow clients to use their own coping mechanisms (information found in the strength-oriented nursing record), use flexible medication orders, and reposition the clients frequently and gently. The mutual goal should be comfort. When pain medication is given and how much pain relief clients get (do they want the edge taken off the pain so they can still be alert, or do they want to sleep for a while) should be the clients' decision.

SUMMARY

The well model is applicable to the dying client because care of the dying should not be disease-oriented but whole-client oriented. The whole person is dying, not just his or her weak heart. As difficult as this time is, clients bring to this process a lifetime of experiences. The positive aspects of their lives help them adapt to changes and are growth-producing. The negative aspects do not promote growth or equilibrium.

Just as other clients need to exercise their rights, so dying clients need to remain in control of their lives until the end. The advocate must especially guard clients' rights to (1) knowledge of the truth, (2) confidentiality and privacy, (3) consent to treatment, (4) choice of a place to die and (5) determination of the disposition of their bodies.

Several concepts are essential to the understanding of the care of the dying within a well model framework. Dying is the final crisis of living and as such may require the use of crisis-intervention skills. The nurse can use clients' negative and positive potentials to help them regain their equilibrium during the dying process.

They must experience the partial deaths of a gradually deteriorating illness and grieve in anticipation of future losses. Grief is a dynamic process by which a person adapts to the loss of a valued object. It is characterized by profound sadness and feelings of emptiness. There is no one best way to grieve.

Grief is most frequently identified as a series of stages, but viewing grief as well-defined stages promotes formularizing or pigeonholing of clients. It also implies an invariant normal pattern of emotional and behavioral change. Moreover, it also implies that each nurse should be able to identify the stage and help the client through it. Differences in staging for acute and chronic dying are not mentioned. Finally, stage theory does not consider individual personality styles and coping mechanisms. The major theorists discussed in this chapter are Kübler-Ross, Engle, Lindemann, Weisman, and Gullo.

Body-image change occurs throughout life as a result of maturation and socialization. The dying client also experiences body-image change of often massive proportion. This change may require viewing oneself as almost a different person. The nurse needs to support the client's efforts to adjust to body-image change by giving reassuance that the person is still acceptable.

Pain for some dying clients may make their remaining days a nightmare. We have discussed it in both its cognitive and affective meaning, that is, its relation to perception and to symbolic meanings. Previous experiences with pain and residual feelings about it also affect response. Nurses should support the ways clients usually cope with pain. Some typical coping behaviors are mentioned in Copp's study; they include strenuous work or play, motionlessness, application of heat or cold, and pacing. There is also a need for more flexible medication orders and experimentation in other modalities for treating pain.

Finally, everyone knows today, but tomorrow may be very frightening for the dying person. Will it bring increasing pain, more surgery, death? Who will care for spouse or children? Is there time left to complete unfinished business, such as repairing broken relationships and providing for future financial needs of survivors? No one can imagine not existing. A willingness to be with the person who has all these things to worry about makes the unknown future easier to bear. This is advocacy with the dying.

The next chapter will discuss the care of the acutely dying client. The concepts in Chapter Five are applicable to care of both acutely dying and chronically dying clients.

QUESTIONS FOR REFLECTION AND DISCUSSION

5-1 What are the rights of the terminally ill? How can the nurse as advocate ensure these rights to all terminally ill clients?

5-2 Have you ever experienced any partial deaths or losses in your life? When? How did you handle them?

5-3 Choose a dying client. Does he or she know the diagnosis? If yes, who, when, where, and how was the client told? Does he or she know of its terminality? Ask the person to draw a picture of himself or herself. What do you see in it? Does the family know the diagnosis and the expected terminality? If yes, who, where, when, and how were they told? How is this client meeting maturational tasks while ill?

5-4 What are the characteristics of a crisis? How does dying apply to crisis theory?

5-5 Have you ever experienced a crisis in your life? What were your feelings at the time? How did you cope with the situation? Were these actions effective in reducing anxiety and restoring equilibrium?

5-6 Describe the differences and similarities between anticipatory grief and bereavement.

5-7 In your culture, what are acceptable modes of grieving?

5-8 Compare Engle's and Kübler-Ross's stages of grieving.

5-9 Describe the symptoms of acute grief.

5-10 Describe morbid or pathological grief reactions.

5-11 What is regrief therapy?

5-12 Give an example of middle knowledge. Describe first-, second-, and third-order denial.

5-13 How does body-image change affect the dying client?

5-14 What are some symbolic meanings of pain?

5-15 What is vigilant focusing, and how is it used as a pain response?

BIBLIOGRAPHY

Aguilera, D.: "Crisis: Death and Dying," *ANA Clinical Sessions*, New York, Appleton-Century-Crofts, 1968.

———, and Messick, J.: *Crisis Intervention, Theory and Methodology*, 2d ed., St. Louis, C. V. Mosby Co., 1974.

Aldrich, C.: "The Dying Patients' Grief," *Journal of American Medical Association*, 184(5):329–331, May 1963.

Annas, G.: *The Rights of Hospital Patients, The Basic ACLU Guide to a Hospital Patient's Rights*, New York, Avon Books, 1975.

———: "Rights of the Terminally Ill Patient," *Journal of Nursing Administration*, 40–44, March-April 1974.

Carlson, C.: "Grief and Mourning," in Carlson, C. (ed.), *Behavioral Concepts and Nursing Intervention*, Philadelphia, J. B. Lippincott Co., 1970.

Copp, L.: "The Spectrum of Suffering," *American Journal of Nursing*, 74(3):491–495, March 1974.

Corbeil, M.: "Nursing Process for a Patient with a Body Image Disturbance," *The Nursing Clinics of North America* 6(1):155–163, March 1971.

Eissler, K.: *Psychiatrist and Dying Patient*, New York, International Universities Press, 1955.

Engle, G.: "Is Grief a Disease?" *Psychosomatic Medicine*, 23(1):18–22, 1961.

———: *Psychological Development in Health and Disease*, Philadelphia, J. B. Lippincott Co., 1962.

Gullo, S., et al.: "Suggested Stages and Response Styles in Life Threatening Illness: A Focus on the Cancer Patient," in Schoenberg, B., et al. (eds.), *Anticipatory grief*, New York, Columbia University Press, 1974.

Hitchcock, J.: "Crisis Intervention, the Pebble in the Pool," *American Journal of Nursing*, 73(8):1388–1390, August 1973.

Hollis, E. R.: "Law Goes into Effect in California Giving the Terminally Ill the Right to Die by Barring Medical Aid," *New York Times*, January 2, 1977.

Jacobson, G., et al.: "Generic and Individual Approaches to Crisis Intervention," *American Journal of Public Health*, 58:339–342, 1968.

Kübler-Ross, E.: *On Death and Dying*, New York, Macmillan Co., 1969.

———: "On the Use of Psychopharmacologic Agents for the Dying Patient and the Bereaved," *The Journal of Thanatology*, 2(1–2): 563–566, Winter–Spring 1972.

Kuenzi, S., and Fenton, M.: "Crisis Intervention in Acute Care Areas," *American Journal of Nursing*, 75(5):830–834, May 1975.

Lindemann, E.: "Symptomatology and Management of Acute Grief," *American Journal of Psychiatry*, 101:141–148, September 1944.

McLachlan, E.: "Recognizing Pain," *American Journal of Nursing*, 74(3):496–497, March 1974.

Murray, J.: "Psychology of the Pain Experience," *The Journal of Psychology*, 78:193–206, July 1971.

Murray, R.: "Principles of Nursing Intervention for the Adult Patient with Body Image Changes," *The Nursing Clinics of North America*, 7(4):677–707, December 1972.

Norris, C.: "The Professional Nurse and Body Image," in Carlson, C. (ed.), *Behavioral Concepts and Nursing Intervention*, Philadelphia, J. B. Lippincott Co., 1970.

Peretz, D.: "Development, Object-Relationships, and Loss," in Schoenberg, B., et al. (eds.), *Loss and Grief: Psychological Management in Medical Practice*, New York, Columbia University Press, 1970.

——: "Reaction to Loss," in Schoenberg, B., et al. (eds.), *Loss and Grief: Psychological Management in Medical Practice*, New York, Columbia University Press, 1970.

Phillips, L.: *Human Adaptation and Its Failures*, New York, Academic Press, 1968.

Rapaport, L.: "The State of Crisis: Some Theoretical Considerations," in Parad, H. (ed.), *Crisis Intervention, Selected Readings*, New York, Family Service Association of America, 1965.

Sadler, A., et al.: "The Uniform Anatomical Gift Act, A Model of Reform," *Journal of American Medical Association*, 206(11):2505–2506, December 9, 1968.

Saunders, C.: "A Therapeutic Community: St. Christopher's Hospice," in Schoenberg, B., et al. (eds.), *Psychosocial Aspects of Terminal Care*, New York, Columbia University Press, 1972.

Schmale, A.: "Normal Grief Is Not a Disease," *Journal of Thanatology*, 2(3–4):807–813, Summer–Fall 1972.

Shneidman, E.: *Deaths of Man*, Baltimore, Penguin Books, 1974.

Siegele, D.: "The Gate Control Theory," *American Journal of Nursing*, 74(3):498–502, May 1974.

Stephens, G.: "Mind-Body Continuum in Human Sexuality," *American Journal of Nursing*, 70(7):1468–1471, July 1970.

Tarasuk, M., et al.: "An Experimental Test of the Importance of Communication Skills for Effective Nursing," in Skipper, J., and Leonard, R., (eds.), *Social Interaction and Patient Care*, Philadelphia, J. B. Lippincott Co., 1965.

Taves, I: *Love Must Not Be Wasted; When Sorrow Comes Take It Gently by the Hand*, New York, Thomas Y. Crowell Co., 1974.

Volkan, V.: "More on Re-Grief Therapy," *Journal of Thanatology*, 3(2):77–91, 1975.

Weisman, A.: *On Dying and Denying, A Psychiatric Study of Terminality*, New York, Behavioral Publications, 1972.

Zind, R.: "Deterrants to Crisis Intervention in the Hospital Unit," *The Nursing Clinics of North America*, 9(1):27–36, March 1974.

Chapter 6

Care of the Acutely Dying

When discussing care of the dying, the diagnosis that usually comes to mind is cancer. However, the primary cause of death in the United States is heart disease. Heart disease can be a chronic problem, or it can bring death in a few minutes, hours, or days. People also die quickly from many other conditions, such as accidents, burns, pancreatitis, gastrointestinal hemorrhage, and ruptured aneurysms, to name a few. Therefore, nursing the dying is more than nursing the cancer client.

The time factor is a crucial determinant of the kind of care given the dying client. This chapter is directed specifically toward the nurse who is working in acute care settings, such as intensive care units, emergency rooms, or other areas of the hospital where a client may suddenly, "take a turn for the worse" and die within a short time without being transferred to the intensive care unit.

Some of the needs of acutely dying clients are the same as those of chronically dying clients. However, the brief time available makes the acutely dying client's needs that much more imperative and poignant. Also, some of these needs may be different by virtue of the nature of the illness and the environment. Pervading all kinds of acute illnesses and various settings is the potential for an actual crisis situation.

Whether or not the family in an acute care setting perceives the client as dying, the situation is fraught with hazard. Anxiety is high. Even if nurses are not aware that a family is grieving, they must at least understand that the family is extremely concerned and anxious.

For nurses, conflict is implied by the essential nature of the situation. They work in the hospital setting to restore life, not to help a client die peacefully, but the setting itself provides daily reminders of life threats and actually the frequency of death is much higher in these settings. "The highest contact with dying patients occurs in ICU/CCU, emergency, medical/surgical, and geriatrics in that order. The lowest contact in Ob/Gyn, psychiatry, and pediatrics."* In-service education of intensive care unit and emergency ward nurses includes all the technical and physiological aspects of care and almost no attention to clients', families', or nurses' emotional needs in these highly volatile settings. Everyone involved with the acutely dying client is in an actual or potential crisis situation. For these reasons and many others, this chapter also discusses nurses' conflicts in the acute care setting.

TEMPORAL-ENVIRONMENTAL CONDITIONS

The setting and its level of activity can have an effect on the client's reactions and adjustment. A coronary care unit is usually a quiet but tension-filled environment with periods of frenzied activity during which the alert client may sense an element of tension in the quiet calmness. By virtue of physical closeness, the coronary client can see and hear any and all resuscitation efforts. An interesting finding in Hackett et al.'s study of psychological hazards in coronary care unit found the following:

> The initial response to watching the arrest was irritability and annoyance . . . rapidly followed by astonishment at the efficiency of the arrest team. All who witnessed the event described the activity with remarkable clarity. Sounds and imagination must have been involved because most accounts came through as if the bed curtain had not been drawn . . . although empathy for the victim was expressed by all . . . none identified himself with the patient affected.†

Not only resuscitative measures can be witnessed, but other emergency situations, such as seizures and hemorrhages, are visible to the clients.

In contrast, the intensive care unit with, for example, respiratory, neurological, and surgical clients or even a recovery room—is usually bustling with activity. The turnover rate of clients is high, with some dying and others being transferred to other floors. Bright lights may shine around the clock. In various stages of alertness, many clients observe other clients more and less seriously

*D. Popoff et al., "What Are Your Feelings about Death and Dying, Part I," *Nursing 75*, **5**(8):17, August 1975.

†T. Hackett et al., "The Coronary Care Unit, An Appraisal of Its Psychologic Hazards," *The New England Journal of Medicine*, **279**(25):1367, December 19, 1968.

ill than themselves. Both sexes are frequently kept in the same open ward. Sometimes clients' bodies are exposed because the nurse forgets to close the curtain when care is being given. Physical space is usually compact and filled with many kinds of machines and equipment.

DEFINITION OF ACUTELY DYING

For want of a better definition, *acutely dying persons* can be said to expire within a few hours or days after onset of the illness. For some, such as the accident victim, death comes after a couple of weeks of vigorous treatment. Any definition of acutely dying must encompass the entire situation, including the nature of the illness, the staff's awareness of the dying trajectory, and efforts made to restore health. Of course, such a definition can be made only after the fact, since clients who have been expected to die within hours sometimes live for years.

CLIENTS' REACTIONS

The factors determining a client's reactions to the acutely dying situation are too numerous to mention here. Some of the contributing variables include nature of the illness, setting, preillness personality, and intrapsychic coping mechanisms.

The nature of the illness can vary from the case of a dying mother or infant in an obstetrical setting, to a car accident victim in the coronary care unit, or to a client in the surgical intensive care unit or recovery room dying of a neurological insult. But the one common denominator is the reality of imminent life threat. In these various situations, clients' awareness of their condition and environment is variable, the coronary client probably being most alert and the client in the emergency ward, surgical intensive care unit, or recovery room least alert.

In a state of emotional and physical disequilibrium, clients focus attention primarily on their immediate needs and environment. They require immediate gratifications of comfort needs and symptom relief. Simultaneously they have many unpleasant feelings, physical distress, heavy medication, and diminished alertness. They are immobilized both by their illness or injury and by being attached to machines. Some clients must be gradually removed from the machines because they have become psychologically dependent upon them. This equipment and intrusive strangers increase clients' feelings of fear, helplessness, and isolation. They lose all sense of personal space; all that is familiar to them is left outside the walls of the ward. Because of the constant attention they may lose hours of sleep and sensorily may be overloaded or deprived.

Even though less than sentient, they may question and recognize the real possibility of death in the near future due to failure of their physiochemical processes or mechanical problems. Above all, the acute care setting reinforces complete dependence upon the omnipotent doctors and nurses. Attention to physical care often deflects attention from emotional needs, mostly eliminating clients' opportunity to express needs and fears and to ask questions.

For the dying client, acute care settings are not established for comfort care but rather for rigorous treatment for survival. Cure care is quite different from comfort care. The inconvenience, discomfort, and sometimes pain of many treatments and machines is a small price to pay for survival, but the inevitably and imminently dying client needs comfort, and intensive care units are not places for comfort.

From a well model perspective acutely dying clients are in a state of extreme disequilibrium. Negative potentials may appear to outweigh positive potentials. The presence of the family should be supported as a positive potential. The staff should attempt to minimize negative potentials, for instance, by administering vasopressor agents for hypotension. The negative potential of loneliness, depersonalization, and fright can be ameliorated by communication efforts of staff and family. The mutual unstated goal is survival, and all efforts are expended in that direction.

COPING MECHANISMS

Some research has been done on reactions to acute life-threatening illness, for example, myocardial infarction. While one cannot generalize from the studies, they are noteworthy and do add to our meager understanding of what it is like to experience an imminent life threat. Gullo et al. identify several coping styles in life-threatening illness (see Chapter 5). In brief they are death-accepter, death-submitter, death-denier, death-defier, and death-transcender. As long as these coping patterns continue to be effective, these same patterns will be used over and over again. It is not predictable, though, that because the client used a specific coping pattern for many years it will continue to be used in the current situation; previous coping patterns may not meet current needs.

Lazarus has identified two major reaction patterns for coping with any threat which are applicable to the acutely dying situation: (1) action tendencies aimed at eliminating or mitigating the anticipated harmful confrontation''*; that is, the acutely dying client cooperates with health care personnel in an institution where restoration of life and health can be found; (2) "cognitive maneuvers through which appraisal is altered without action directed at changing the objective situation''†; in other words, defense mechanisms are used by the acutely dying client to minimize the threat of loss and to allow maximum functioning under these extreme circumstances.

Many people believe Kübler-Ross's stages of dying to be an accurate picture of the psychological adaptation to dying in all time frames. However,

---

*R. Lazarus, *Psychological Stress and the Coping Process*, New York, McGraw-Hill Book Co., 1966, p. 258.
†Ibid., p. 259.

her findings were based on a study of chronically dying clients, for whom time was available to ruminate about their lives and losses. Acutely dying clients do not have this time, and their unique problems and reactions have yet to be adequately investigated.

Although such a thorough study on acutely dying clients is not as yet available, insight can be gained from the reactions of clients who have experienced a life threat during an acute illness. Often it is impossible to tell during a very critical situation whether the client is viable or in fact dying. Many times the act of dying is recognized in retrospect. Therefore it is the responsibility of the nurse (1) to recognize the critical nature of an acute illness, (2) to acknowledge the potential for death, and (3) to allow the client to use whatever mechanisms are necessary to maintain some equilibrium in a very unstable and deteriorating situation. The point is not to decide that a particular mechanism is "pathological" but to recognize that severe stress is behind the emergency coping mechanisms.

In terms of the well model, these coping mechanisms may be looked upon as positive potentials since they help to maintain a sense of integrity. However, when the coping mechanisms seriously compromise the efforts of the staff to care for the client, these mechanisms become negative potentials.

Hamburg et al. cite an example of an emergency defense mechanism, denial, in a burned client:

> Patient B . . . died two weeks after injury. . . . although she preferred not to think about . . . the injury . . . she remembered it clearly. However, within a few days she developed the attitude that she was not seriously ill at all, but practically well. She then recalled having been afraid of dying immediately after the injury. . . . She asserted that she was not helpless, but to a considerable extent could care for herself. . . . The fact that this patient made such statements calmly and deliberately while she lay helplessly on a Stryker frame—a charred remnant of a woman—had a powerful impact on all observers.*

It was necessary for patient B to so blatantly deny the seriousness of her burn in view of the serious life threat she was experiencing. The threat was too great for her to handle; therefore she could not acknowledge it. (See Figure 6-1.)

Initial Impact of an Acute Life-Threatening Situation

The shock of a critical illness or injury requires a strong reaction from the client aimed to minimized threat or loss, in other words, to maintain equilibrium. The anxiety level is extremely high and proportional to the perception of life threat. Anxiety can also be free-floating in that everything may be a source of extreme concern. Anxiety forms the basis for other behavioral responses.

In addition to anxiety the client has a sense of depersonalization, including

*D. Hamburg et al., "Adaptive Problems and Mechanisms in Severely Burned Patients," *Psychiatry, The Journal of the Study of Interpersonal Processes*, **16**(9):1, February 1953.

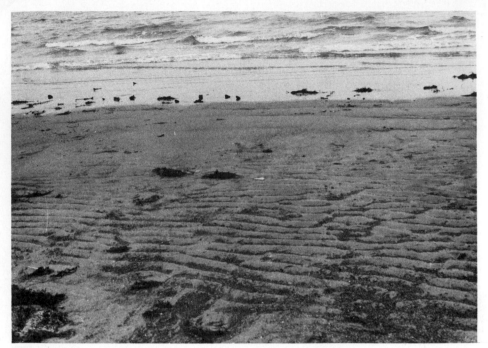

Figure 6-1 As water ripples sand, pain scars the flesh and the spirit.

a sense of numbness, strangeness, and unreality. Nurses must be aware of clients' anxiety and sense of depersonalization, be willing to spend extra time with the clients, listen carefully, and find ways to reassure them. Nurses must try to find out who a client is as a person. Roberts suggests several ways nurses can foster personalization in the critical care setting. Upon admission an exchange of names is important, as is orienting clients to the new surroundings. Good eye and tactile contact also helps to personalize. All diagnostic tests and procedures should be explained in a relaxed manner as much as possible. Clients should be given choices in care. Family visits and having some small personal objects on the bedside table give them a sense of continuity with the healthy self beyond the crisis environment. Nurses should also try to empathize with clients.

Hackett et al. observed that 40 out of 50 clients in the coronary care unit exhibit overtly anxious behaviors. High levels of anxiety have also precipitated and increased mortality rates from heart attack.

In burned clients, Hamburg et al. (corroborated later by Schlichtmann) cite emergency defense mechanisms extending from the time of injury to the time the physiological emergency is over, sometimes lasting weeks. All the mechanisms were used at various times by clients. Although Hamburg did not stage these emergency mechanisms, this period of time is comparable to Engle's first stage of loss, that of shock and disbelief. (See Chapter 5 for a fuller description of Engle's stages of adaptation to loss.)

Emergency Defense Mechanisms

1 *Constriction*   The client exhibits a flat affect with tight control over recognition and expression of all emotions, often with an attitude of resignation.

2 *Suppression*   The client makes a conscious effort to avoid thinking about the unpleasant experience.

3 *Repression*   The client unconsciously excludes the affect associated with a remembered trauma: the expression.

4 *Denial*   The client rejects some obvious aspect of reality, either the injury or its consequences.

5 *Delusion, illusion, and hallucination formation*   The client distorts reality to a greater degree than denial. Both Hamburg and Schlichtmann cited delusion, illusion, and hallucination as a worsening of clients' physical condition; clients subsequently died.

6 *Regression*   The client became extremely demanding, complaining, attention-seeking, and dependent in relationships.

7 *Reworking*   In an effort to decrease anxiety the client repetitively reviews the traumatic experience.

8 *Withdrawal*   The client becomes shy, avoids people, and resorts to fantasy. (This occurred only in the first 2 weeks with a very few clients. For the most part clients were very responsive to contact with others.)

9 *Religiosity*   The client becomes philosophical and resigned to the injury. (Religiosity is not used in a spiritual sense but in a more fatalistic or philosophical sense.)

10 *Rationalization*   The client has a need to justify dependence, hostility, or irresponsibility.

11 *Conversion*   The client develops physical symptoms to meet a covert need.

The nature of the injury determines the length of time clients remain in the acute phase of illness and therefore uses emergency defense mechanisms. For example, the client with a myocardial infarction has a shorter acute phase than the burn victim.

Specifically, the client with a myocardial infarction may exhibit four brood behavioral responses as identified by Scalzi: (1) Anxiety is manifested by increased verbalization, inability to concentrate, understand or retain information, restlessness or insomnia, muscular rigidity, palmar sweating, tremulousness, and tachycardia. (2) Denial is manifested by history of ignoring symptoms prior to admission, avoiding discussion of heart attack or its meaning, or minimizing its severity or consequences. In addition clients describe their condition by quoting others and not expressing their own opinion, or they intellectually acknowledge their heart attack but emotionally disregard it by ignoring the therapeutic regimen. They also can be overtly cheerful and socially humorous in verbal interactions, and may "shop around" for a suitable answer to their questions by asking some questions of several staff members. (3) Corresponding to Engle's second stage, when reality sets in, depression is manifested after the first 2 to 3 days by a sad, listless look, disinterest, and expressions of pessimism or hopelessness. Clients give minimal verbal responses, display slowness in movement and speech, and withdraw by sleeping more and drawing the curtains. They frequently become anorexic, cry, and express direct and projected anger. (4) Clients may fear a threat to sexual adequacy, attractiveness, and ability. Therefore, they may exhibit aggressive sexual behavior to compensate for this perceived loss of ability and attractiveness. They may make seductive or flirtatious comments and compliments and attempt to hold, fondle, or kiss parts of the nurse's body. They may also deliberately expose their genitals and boast about their past sexual interest and prowess.

THE NEEDS OF THE ACUTELY DYING CLIENT

All dying clients have some basic needs. The nursing process is used to identify, plan, meet, and evaluate these needs. Assessment was discussed in Chapter 4 and provides the guidelines to meet these needs. Three basic things are required of the nurse: (1) recognition of existence of needs, (2) client approval, or at least absence of client disapproval (because of the nature of the illness some clients cannot assent to care), and (3) decision on priorities.

In terms of the well model these needs are neither negative nor positive potentials. When these needs are met adequately either by the client alone or with the help of someone else, they become positive potentials that help to maintain a sense of adequacy and wholeness even in a very unstable, rapidly deteriorating condition. The threat of or actual loss of a part of the healthy self is a negative potential to which the nurse and other members of the health team must address themselves. Even during the dying trajectory, clients' needs are potentials for growth. The seemingly contradictory concept of growth in dying can be seen in meeting dying clients' needs.

How these needs are met depends upon the time available, appropriate personnel, and a place in which to meet these needs. For acutely dying clients some modification of the basic nursing process is necessary. For instance, in planning to meet acutely dying clients' needs, time may not be available for a team conference or preparation of a Kardex for continuity of care. Planning by necessity must be quick and at times noncollaborative or independent, but every effort should be made to provide good care while considering the person who is dying and not violating any of his or her legal and human rights.

The following paragraphs discuss the needs of acutely dying clients. They are not presented in any particular order of importance but are complementary and must be considered as a whole. Each need affects the others, but priorities change as, during the dying trajectory, needs shift and assume increasing or decreasing importance.

Communication

Even acutely dying clients are social beings, but their degree of alertness determines how the nurse, staff, and family try to communicate with them. It is part of the nurse's role to help clients maintain contact with their environment. Many studies have been done describing the deleterious effects of either sensory deprivation or overload.

Unconscious clients still may be able to hear. The nurse's physical presence may be sensed. Explaining to unconscious clients, even in the flurry of physical activity, who you are, where they are, what is the matter, and what is being done for them is necessary to reduce anxiety. Touch is also an important method of communication even with unconscious clients, as evidenced by Kreiger's studies. Thus, even if clients are unconscious the staff should not make grim prognostications of their hopeless condition in their presence. With effort and interest, a nurse can acquire a level of sensitivity to clients that does not require verbal communication. In the true sense of the words the nurse then is "anticipating the client's needs." Some nurses develop a sensitivity to subtle physical changes in clients before noticeable objective signs are apparent.

When clients are conscious the nurse should speak to them. The nurse should observe clients' body language, for example, the degree of tension exhibited in a clenched fist or frightened eyes, and should not walk away if a client is anxious or in any other way trying to communicate. Soothing words from a nurse have little meaning when not supported by actions. Physical touch is very reassuring to most people. The client who is conscious but unable to communicate fully and coherently is a challenge to the nurse. Some of the reasons for inadequate communication may be the pathophysiology of the illness, such as neurological insult, poor vision, or faulty hearing; tracheotomy; oxygen mask; restrained hands; and heavy medication. Sensory deprivation is thought to be a major problem in "ICU psychosis."

Glaser and Strauss have found that usually nurses adjust their emotional involvement and interaction depending upon clients' awareness of their terminal condition. The more uncomfortable nurses feel, the less involvement and contact there are. There are four basic types of awareness:

1 *Closed awareness*   The client is not told of impending death although the nurse knows; the client speaks freely but the nurse is guarded in conversation.

2 *Suspicion awareness*   The client suspects he or she is going to die but the doctor has not told the person yet. While this is a contest for control, the client does not ask directly. This is an unstable situation.

3 *Mutual pretence*   Both nurse and client know the client is going to die, but prefer not to talk about it. This is also a very unstable situation and conversation is carefully guarded.

4 *Open awareness*   Both the client and nurse know the fatal outcome and acknowledge it as such.

These awareness contexts occur with all dying clients.

Every effort must be made to identify clients' needs. In addition, it is even possible that the clients will ask if they are dying. There is no one right answer to this question. The situation and the people involved must determine the answer. The balance between realism and hope is very difficult to achieve and maintain in an acutely dying situation. Kübler-Ross suggests that in the acute situation, clients should not be told they are dying but should be told that they are seriously ill but everyone is working very hard to help them recover.

Moreover, in the emergency room it is important to be discrete in telling a critically ill or injured client of the death of a family member, passenger, or victim.

Because clients are in a strange and frightening environment, the family's presence helps them maintain a sense of the familiar and avoid the feeling of abandonment so many dying clients fear. Unfortunately most families are sent to the waiting room while life saving care is being given. That is not to suggest that the family be present as a client is being defibrillated or while massive bleeding is evident. However, efforts should be made to allow the family more visiting time.

The following guidelines are helpful in maintaining clients' communication:

1   Do not say anything in the presence of clients that you do not want them to hear.
2   Offer them imformation about who you are, where they are, and what is happening.
3   Do not tell clients they are dying. Offer words of encouragement, such as "We are working very hard to help you."
4   Encourage the family to stay nearby.
5   Do not abandon clients or family.

Positive Body Image

To acutely dying clients, body-image change and adaptation is not relevant. They retain their previous, pretrauma body image. Change in body image is a gradual process. Acutely dying clients would be in the state of shock and disbelief in Engle's stages of adaptation to loss (see Figure 5-3). Denial of the impact is an apparently necessary coping mechanism. In addition, the clients may also exhibit despair, discouragement, and passive acceptance.

The nurse may be totally ineffective in presenting the reality of physical change to clients, because they are probably not ready to absorb it, but the clients may request an explanation of what has happened. The only recourse is to answer honestly.

Physical Care

Most books about pychological care of clients ignore physical care aspects, but the acutely dying need physical care as well as psychological care. The nurses working in acute care settings are experts on physical care. Machines have become the extension of the nurse's arm. Intravenous, medication, and dietary therapy are necessary adjuncts to such comfort measures as turning and bathing. The point when physical curative care changes to physical comfort care and palliation is very difficult to define.

Control over the Environment

In a weak, completely dependent position, clients have no control over themselves or their environment. They may even be unable to express their wishes.

There are a few things which can be done to provide clients with a renewed sense of control over their environment. These guidelines are general.

1   Allow clients choices in their care.
2   Explain all treatments and the need for them.
3   Restrain clients only when absolutely necessary, and then give a full explanation.

Self-esteem

Feelings of self-worth are closely related to control over environment and communication. Clients who sense they have no control over themselves or their environment feel lowered self-esteem. In the acutely dying situation clients need to be reassured that everything necessary is being done for them by competent people.

A few guidelines are suggested to help them maintain self-esteem:

1   Do not avoid the clients.
2   Give them information about what is happening.
3   Answer questions honestly.
4   Encourage family visiting.

Opportunity to Grieve for Themselves

Just as body-image change takes place over time, so does resolution of grief. Acutely dying clients may have no time to grieve for themselves. Their only reaction to realization of imminent death may be fright. (See the section in Chapter 5 on grief and loss for further discussion.)

The following guidelines will help acutely dying clients grieve:

1   Encourage verbalization of feelings, especially crying and anger.
2   Observe nonverbal behavior indicating anxiety.

Opportunity for a Life Review

Closely related to the need to grieve is dying clients' need for a life review. The life review is the reminiscence of accomplishments and failures in their lives. Again, acutely dying clients are short-changed in fulfilling their needs. Time is not available, except in instances after a close call with death.

This guideline will encourage life review:

1   Allow clients to talk about themselves.

Relief from Pain

Acutely dying clients have an immediate need for pain relief. This fright and physical distress only add to the perception of pain. Time may not be available to learn clients' pain history or usual responses to pain. Verbal expressions of pain and requests for pain relief may not be possible.

The nurse must be alert to nonverbal cues in clients. Pain triggers an increased sympathetic nervous system response and production of epinephrine, causing tachycardia, increased cardiac output, and peripheral vasoconstriction, which may increase blood pressure. "Such changes can be life-threatening to the patient who is hypertensive or has had a recent myocardial infarction."* Additional physiological changes in response to pain perception include respiratory changes, excessive perspiration, nausea and vomiting, and skin color changes. Muscular changes include local or generalized rigidity, writhing, unusual postures such as knees bent up to abdomen, restlessness, rubbing, and scratching. Sensorium changes include excitement, irritability, depression, unusual quietness, withdrawal, behavior reversals, and increasing disorientation.

A few guidelines will help in keeping clients as pain-free as possible.

1 Give medication on time. Do not keep clients waiting without a good explanation.
2 Monitor clients responses to medication.
3 Do any painful treatments when medication provides the most relief.
4 Encourage clients to use their own coping responses to pain.

Spiritual Comfort

It seems appropriate to end this list of needs of acutely dying clients with a most fundamental need for many clients. The most common response, of course, to meeting spiritual needs of clients, especially in a crisis situation, is to (1) find out what religion the person espouses and (2) call a member of the clergy.

Even in the acutely ill situation there is much more a nurse can do.

In defining the spiritual needs of clients Sister Corita Dickinson's definition of spiritual aspects of nursing applies: "The spiritual aspects of nursing . . . are linked to a hope for survival and a search for meaning in all experiences, including illness."† The spiritual aspects of nursing, then, are much more than the traditional religious experience. They bring out the therapeutic use of self and a commitment to and respect for the dying person. When I have had the opportunity to care for a dying person I feel profoundly touched and experience a sense of privilege and humility to have known that person even for a very brief time. For there is a strength in vulnerability for both the client and the nurse. Although nurses are not accountable for spiritual care in an institutional sense, as they are for numbers of bed baths or injections, it is an essential part of total client care.

These guidelines will be helpful in assisting clients to meet their spiritual needs:

1 Listen carefully to clients' expression of their beliefs.

*E. McLachlin, "Recognizing Pain," *American Journal of Nursing*, **74**(3):497, March 1974.
†Sister C. Dickinson, "The Search for Spiritual Meaning," *American Journal of Nursing*, **75**(10):1971, October 1975.

2   Allow clients time to be alone to reflect.
3   If clients wish, encourage clergy visits.

FAMILY'S REACTION

The family waits and waits for news, and the waiting seems endless. Although nurses do believe they should support families in acute care units, in practice the families may get short shrift. The demands of caring for the client sometimes leave little energy to consider the family's needs. With the exception of the comatose client's family, a nurse's interaction with the family is not as frequent with the client.

In an acute care setting, whether or not the family perceives the client as dying, the situation is hazardous; they feel helpless and frightened. This anxiety precipitates several kinds of difficult situations. Anger may be free-floating and directed at anyone or anything. The family is simultaneously living with the reality of the client's immediate needs and dealing with the question of the person's future survival. Even in the waiting area of an emergency room, only brief visits may be allowed. A nurse who is unaware that the family is grieving should at least understand that the family is extremely concerned about the client.

Both family and client are forced to rely on the ability and effort of the nurses and doctors to sustain life. Unable to adequately evaluate the quality of care from a medical standpoint, the family's only criteria are the quality of interpersonal communication with the nurse and the physical details of care, especially comfort measures.

First, they want to visit as often as possible. In the acute care setting, the hospital policy usually allows one or two visitors for 5 minutes every hour. The visiting hours should be more flexible to accommodate the family's and client's need to be together. When dying is imminent the family should be allowed to stay in the room.

Second, families often ask the same questions every hour, such as seeking information about blood pressure or temperature for example. An attitude of courteous, warm concern should be conveyed by the staff to family members at all times. It is advisable to offer information even if it is not hopeful. In the acute setting, especially with so little preparation, the family needs to know the facts so that the inevitability of the death becomes a reality.

Because of a family's state of mild panic, members may not be able to hear the answers to questions or they may focus on one or two words and phrases and distort the meaning. With increasing anxiety, the family's focus of interest narrows sharply. Its priorities may be very different from the nurse's. The family, for example, may be concerned about comfort measures, such as keeping the client's face free of perspiration or changing blood-splattered sheets, while the nurse is trying to maintain a patent airway. To family members, comfort measures indicate good nursing care, and the discrepancy between what the family feels should be done and what is done will decrease confidence in care and increase anxiety. Because of its anxiety level the family sometimes has difficulty in understanding the need for uncomfortable and sometimes painful treatments. Sometimes family members feel better if they can help by doing some small task such as giving a drink of water or helping to wash the client. These activities should be encouraged.

Third, the family's need for information when not visiting may precipitate numerous lengthy telephone calls, interrupting care and tying up the telephone at the nurses' station. Making standard replies such as "no change" or requesting the telephone operator not to allow the calls through to the nurses' station are sometimes necessary in extreme situations.

Four, there are other factors that add to the family's high anxiety level. Both family and client have been thrust into a strange environment with little personal privacy. They also experience a loss of control and an almost total isolation of the client. Eating and sleeping patterns are disrupted. In addition, family members have no place to relax or express grief after leaving the client's bedside. Outside circumstances, for instance, other or recent experiences with family members' dying or being seriously ill, or family members such as children or aged parents being left at home, may also be a source of real concern.

After the death families need much support. The physician should tell the family of the death, so family members do not think the deceased received inadequate medical attention. Family members should never be told of the death in a large public hallway or in a room with other people. Tact and sensitivity are needed by any health team member who assists the family after death. Permission should always be granted to view the body, but staff should remove all tubes and make the body as presentable as possible beforehand, especially in the emergency room after a mutilating accident. Viewing the body immediately after death facilitates the grief process. The family should never be rushed into leaving and should be allowed to sit with the deceased for a few minutes. Cultural expressions of grief should be encouraged. Generally family members should not be sedated because drugs tend to supress normal grief reactions. The person who sits with the family immediately after the death should encourage expressing of feelings. Sometimes it is helpful for someone on the staff to be with a family when details about the autopsy permissions, identification of the body, and funeral and burial arrangements are made. Tact, sensitivity, and warm concern are the hallmarks of the person best qualified to assist at this time.

When summoning the family upon the death of a relative, the staff should never tell relatives over the telephone that the client has died. They should instead convey the seriousness of the situation as well as a sense of urgency. The nurse should be waiting for the relatives' arrival.

Follow-up visits about a month after the death should be a regular part of the continuing care of the family. Encouraging the family to revisit the acute care setting where the death occurred will facilitate the grief process. Many of the same questions will be asked by family members, but now they may be able to hear the answers.

NURSES' REACTIONS

Nurses working with dying clients are under stress. They are expected to provide comfort and care for the clients in a professional manner, but for many nurses, professionalism is still equated with coldness and aloofness. This view of professionalism is counterproductive to the care of the dying. Even if nurses intellectually reject the cold, professional attitude as inappropriate, they may need to withdraw from clients defensively.

Of the many attitudes nurses assume, one of the most prominent is that of the healer and sometimes the omnipotent one. What nurse who has worked hard but unsuccessfully to save a life does not feel let down—bursting that bubble of omnipotence?

Feifel feels that a person entering the medical profession does so with more fear of death than the average person. Could this also be true of nurses? Do physicians and nurses develop a sense of omnipotence to counterbalance the fear of death?

Working in the emotionally charged environment of the dying client, nurses need support and understanding if they are to continue to be helpful to present and future clients.

For the nurse, concern is present and future-oriented, with short-and long-term goals. Present concern for the client's immediate needs and future concern for eventual cure present a care-cure conflict for the nurse. In addition to caring for physiological needs the nurse should (1) recognize when a client may be dying and (2) understand the dying process from both a psychological and a physiological focus. Depending upon the perceived dying trajectory, Glaser and Strauss point out that nurses use different strategies of care and communication. In general, as death draws nearer, interaction is reduced and emotional involvement is diminished. This is even more difficult in the acutely dying setting. As the client nears death, lifesaving treatment may be intensified so that contact with the client is increased and the threat to the nurse is greater.

Grief work is not part of the nurse's job description, but it is an inevitable occurrence in places where clients die. In the specialized acute setting the nurses are especially vulnerable, for they see themselves as healers and get their satisfaction from restoring seriously ill clients to health. They do not view themselves as morticians or keepers of cadavers, although many of their clients are comatose. They may even resent a client admitted to the unit who is very old or obviously terminally ill, as with end-stage hepatic coma or cancer. Nurses do not work with open heart surgery clients to ease their way to a peaceful death. The nature of the therapeutic plan is such that death is unacceptable. Nurses use their technical skills to restore health to very sick clients. So in the acute intensive care setting, they are faced with the paradox that, on the one hand, their highly skilled techniques are used to restore health and, on the other hand, the situation is such that probability of death is greater because of the seriousness of illness.

In acute care settings, nurses are frequently on a one-to-one basis with their clients and must focus their attention on the repetitive, fast-paced details of care. Concentrating on the client, nurses are expected to be objective and perform often uncomfortable, painful, or otherwise anxiety-producing treatments. At the same time they are expected to relieve pain, be compassionate, and ease loneliness and fright.

The turnover of clients in the acute care setting is rapid and allows little time to get to know a client or to experience object loss. Individualized client care is made more difficult by some clients' impaired communicative ability due to decreased consciousness, weakness, or physical obstructions such as tracheotomy. The client who is less than sentient receives minimal or poor psychological care because it is easier to withdraw from an uncommunicative client than from one who is alert and asking for help. In summary, the rapid turnover of clients, the focus on technical care, and the communication problems render adequate psychological care all but impossible at times.

Even though psychological needs may be recognized, they cannot be met. The nurse may feel threatened by clients' coping behaviors such as removing monitor leads, demanding constant attention, being sexually aggressive, crying, and asking questions about death or diagnosis.

In addition to the stress of client needs the nurse may experience some environmental stress, such as the compact, crowded work areas with inconveniently placed equipment. The nurse is constantly observed by alert clients. Mastery of technical skills especially related to complex machinery and understanding of physiological changes is a formidable challenge compounded and complicated by clients with multiple acute active diagnoses. Physically the nurse is required to do a good deal of lifting, reaching, and bending. Furthermore, there may be large numbers of staff members coming in and out of the unit.

Quint describes the concerns of two nurses working in a coronary care unit, which may well be representative of the kinds of stresses all nurses feel in acute care, high-risk situations:

Increased responsibility for making medical judgments of a serious nature . . . increased concern about making mistakes . . . emotional impact of sudden emergency . . . always the same. Recognition of emergency brought a breathless feeling, like a sudden surge of electrical energy, after which they began to perform the necessary actions almost mechanically. With the end of the emergency . . . a letdown . . . The nurse experiences anxiety, especially . . . her actions mean the difference between life and death . . . the physician . . . also under pressure . . . may express their own tensions by being hypercritical of the nurse . . . The compactness of the unit . . . brings the nurse into close and continuous contact with patients who look directly to her for emotional support as well as treatment. These patients are alert to what is going on, and they watch the nurse's every movement . . . long spans without emergency . . . boredom. At the other extreme there is the emotional exhaustion . . . from losing several patients in a row.*

Possible Solutions

For nurses in the acute care setting to be repeatedly effective, they must nurture a quality of openness and humanness. They must care what happens to their clients. By sharing the psychic pain of their clients, nurses open themselves to hurt. They must be willing to do their own grief work, understanding that it is a necessary, healthy, and restorative process.

The problem of nurses' grief is twofold. First, recognition of nurses' need to grieve—both intellectually and emotionally—must be granted. Second, this need must be legitimized by developing supportive measures on both lateral and vertical planes.

To begin these two steps, both administration and direct care workers must recognize their own humanity and mortality. They must be sympathetic not only to feelings and needs, but also to errors and occasional poor judgments:

We sometimes think we have no right to have anger, sadness, anxiety or despair, probably because our stereotype of a nurse does not picture her with such feelings. We cannot discount the fact, however, that nurses are human beings with all the feelings and fears of average human beings. Just because we became nurses makes us no less persons; we are still individuals.†

In recognizing one's humanity, one needs support at times. Some psychological barriers to seeking this support, as mentioned by Jones, are fears of (1) being ostracized or being considered weak for having certain feelings, (2) being reprimanded by supervisors and colleagues for having negative feelings, (3) being betrayed after revealing very personal feelings, (4) being misunderstood, and (5) having notions about the role of nurses which others share.

To legitimize the need to grieve, support must come from the bureaucratic system and informal, everyday collegial relationships. If nursing is to become more humanistic, it will be necessary for bureaucratic policies, both explicit and implicit, to become more worker-serving than institution-serving.

In addition, it is unrealistic to work for 8 hours (minus a 15-minute coffee break and a 30-minute meal break) giving all acutely ill and dying clients the maximum amount of emotional support needed. If the 8-hour work schedule is a strain, the proposed 10-hour day can only increase the burden and decrease the quality of humanistic care. Although there is very little chance of a major revolution in work patterns in American hospitals, adaptations within the currently used patterns of work hours must realistically be made.

*J. Quint, "The Threat of Death: Some Consequences for Patients and Nurses," *Nursing Forum*, **8**(3):295–296, 1969.

†E. Jones, "Who Supports the Nurse?" *Nursing Outlook*, **10**(7):477, July 1962.

There are several possible ways to provide the needed respite. To legitimize these supports they must be condoned and instituted by the administration. During the workday nurses need time away from the client besides the meal and coffee breaks. This time must be adhered to strictly, or else the tendency to overwork and get overinvolved because of the demands of the job will prevail. A room with some privacy is needed, and not just a bathroom! Many acute care settings, because of the need to observe the client and the compactness of the ward, do not provide a place away from the client and the work of the ward.

Also, nurses need sufficient time off duty to regroup emotional forces. Why should physical illness and somatic complaints be the only legitimate way to take a day off? If nurses are not physically ill but need to get away, they should be allowed to take a mental health day without feeling guilty about it. Better scheduling of rotating shifts with concern for nurses' circadian rhythms would be less fatiguing and more productive. It might also be advantageous to require each staff member to rotate among sections of the hospital on a regular basis for a specific length of time. A different milieu provides a needed change of pace.

Administration should select nurses for acute care settings according to the following criteria: scholastic aptitude, technical expertise, and personal and psychological performance. Sufficient staff should be hired to ensure proper client coverage when nurses are off duty, on holidays or vacations, or out due to illness.

Interpersonal supervisory support, not just policy enforcement, is needed, especially when doubt and fatigue take over. Bernice Harper, Director of the Long Term Care Division of the National Center of Health Resources Administration, has identified several flexible stages of grieving which her social workers go through in caring for a chronically ill dying client. By understanding the need to grieve and providing verbal and nonverbal support through the eventual resolution of the grieving process, Ms. Harper was able to increase the "stay rate" of her workers.* This kind of concern for staff is also necessary in nursing. Ms. Harper in effect affirms the normal grieving process professionals experience, which includes unpleasant feelings. Because of its healing nature, grief provides an opportunity for more insight into oneself, which in turn develops strength to be more human and able to give more of oneself.

In-service education should not focus only on the technical and physiological aspects of client care. Seminars should be planned with clients' and nurses' psychological needs in mind. Group workday meetings with a sensitive person—not necessarily a psychiatrist who is not a direct care giver in the unit and, therefore, is not embroiled in the everyday conflicts in the unit—are helpful. That person, possibly a nurse, should have a background in group dynamics and counseling. These meetings could provide needed mutual support

*B. Harper, Keynote Address on *The Family and Death: A Social Work Symposium*, Foundation of Thanatology, Columbia-Presbyterian Medical Center, New York, April 12, 1975.

on a planned basis. Unplanned but opportune group discussions could also help to air feelings.

On a one-to-one basis, a mutual support system can be very effective. A grieving nurse has a need for support to maintain self-esteem and to mobilize energy. Nurses should always remember that they *share* the responsibility for their clients with other health care personnel even if they are functioning in a primary care setting. That sharing can be done in response to unspoken needs such as behavioral or facial expressions. A shared silence can be very effective. Even in the state of chronic crisis that is the acute care setting, nurses could take time to let the other staff members know they understand by listening to feelings without passing judgment. Nurses should share their own feelings too.

When learning to grieve one also learns more about oneself. Insight into one's limitations and strengths is the growth process through which one becomes a more human person and a more effective nurse. Nurses, for instance, learn the appropriate time for conscious withdrawal from a difficult and overly stressful situation. If fatigue and overconcern are clouding judgment of the client to the point where one refuses to withdraw from the situation, one should ask oneself the following questions: Whose needs are being met in this situation? Have I put the client into an overly dependent position? Am I failing to include other members of the family or health care team who could be helpful?

There is one final kind of support that does not need administrative sanction. Without knowing it, clients can be the support that makes nurses' difficult task of caring for the acutely dying client actually rewarding. The sense or knowledge that one has really helped a client is sometimes sufficient satisfaction for nurses' efforts.

SUMMARY

Dying is usually discussed in terms of chronic care, but many clients die emotionally unprepared in the acute care setting, which exists to restore life. The temporal-environmental conditions determine the kind of care given. Settings in which the customary dying trajectory is rapid, such as coronary and intensive care units and emergency rooms, are open, large, crowded rooms with many kinds of complex machines. Tension pervades the atmosphere. The acutely dying client, by definition, expires in a few hours or days.

Clients react to this setting by feeling threatened, powerless, and stripped of most of their sense of identity and integrity. They can think only of their immediate needs during this crisis. The acute care setting exists to cure and does not provide comfort care for the dying.

A need by itself is neither a negative or a positive potential. It becomes a positive potential when it is adequately met and a negative potential when not adequately met. In terms of the well model, the acutely dying client may appear to have more negative than positive potentials. The client's reactions are dependent on nature of the illness, setting, preillness personality, and intrapsychic coping mechanism. Positive potentials are the client's coping mechanisms. In an emergency clients use many kinds of mental mechanisms and behaviors to reduce this extreme threat. Only when coping mechanisms interfere with care should their effect be minimized.

The nursing process is used to implement and meet acutely dying clients' needs, which are (1) to maintain communication with the environment, (2) to maintain a positive body image in the face of deteriorating physical abilities, (3) to have physical care, (4) to maintain control over one's environment, (5) to maintain self-esteem, (6) to grieve for oneself, (7) to have time for a life review, (8) to have relief from pain, and (9) to have spiritual comfort.

The family is also in crisis. With no preparation the family feels helpless and must rely on the staff for expert care and information. Repetitive questions and frequent visits and telephone calls from the family can be very annoying for staff. On the other hand, normal family life has been suspended while the family waits, and all attention has now been focused on the ill member.

When the member dies families need support immediately and in the near future. Information of the death should always be given in a private place. A staff member, chaplain, or volunteer can be very helpful to the family in several ways. This person can help the grieving process by sitting with family members for awhile, allowing them to view the body immediately after death, helping them make funeral arrangements, and visiting them a month later. A grieving family member should not be sedated since sedation retards the grieving process.

There are many inherent conflicts for nurses in the acutely dying setting. While they work to restore life, they encounter the very sick and even those who are dying. The rapid turnover of clients, the focus on technical care, and the problem of communication with extremely sick clients make comfort care all but impossible. They must help the family, which is also in a state of crisis. Consequently, nurses develop self-protective strategies that diminish their ability to provide humane care. Possible solutions lie in both bureaucratic and collegial psychological measures. Such support for nurses may even increase our stay rate.

The next chapter will discuss problems unique to the chronic care setting, that is, chronically dying clients' needs and nurses' conflicts.

QUESTIONS FOR REFLECTION AND DISCUSSION

6-1   Visit the intensive care unit. Ask the nurses which clients have been identified as dying. What inferences can you make from their response?

6-2   What life-threatening conditions and situations do you observe in the intensive care unit?

6-3   Observe the work of the nurses in the intensive care unit for one shift. Answer the following questions: How many minutes of the day is a nurse out of sight of the client? How long are meal and coffee breaks? Where does the nurse take these breaks? Is paperwork done during meal or coffee break? Is the conversation about clients or about other completely different topics during meal or coffee break? Does the nurse ever get completely away from clients during the workday?

6-4   Ask the nurses in the intensive care unit how they relax at the end of the workday.

6-5   What support mechanisms have been set up for relieving the emotional discomfort of nurses?

6-6   What in-service education did the staff nurse receive to address the interpersonal component of client care in the intensive care unit and emergency room?

6-7   What factors interfere with nurses' providing adequate psychological care to acutely dying clients?

6-8   Identify signs of anxiety of both the client and the family in an intensive care unit and emergency room. Are they using any emergency defense mechanisms?

6-9   What personal items are clients allowed in the intensive care unit? How can the nurse help clients remain in control of their environment?

6-10 What is the rationale for a rotation schedule for nurses in all acute care settings in the hospital? Does it consider the emotional needs of nurses?

6-11 What is the "awareness" context? How does it affect nursing care, in particular, conversation?

6-12 Relate the concept of crisis to the acute care setting. How can a nurse identify a crisis and intervene appropriately in the acute care setting?

6-13 List some ways you avoid your clients.

6-14 How open or visible is death or dying in the acute care setting, and how is it controlled?

6-15 Where are acutely dying clients in the intensive care unit, emergency room, and general medical-surgical unit located spatially?

6-16 In terms of division of labor, who manages the death tasks?

BIBLIOGRAPHY

Benner, P.: "Nurses in the Intensive Care Unit," in Davis, M., et al. (eds.), *Nurses in Practice, A Perspective on Work Environments*, St. Louis, C. V. Mosby Co., 1975.

Bilodeau, C.: "The Nurse and Her Reactions to Critical Care Nursing," *Heart and Lung, The Journal of Critical Care*, 2(3):358–363, May-June 1973.

Cassem, N., and Hackett, T.: "Sources of Tension for the CCU Nurse," *American Journal of Nursing*, 72(8):1426–1430, August 1972.

Caughill, R. (ed.): *The Dying Patient, A Supportive Approach*, Boston, Little, Brown and Co., 1976.

Dickinson, Sister C.: "The Search for Spiritual Meaning," *American Journal of Nursing*, 75(10):1789–1793, October 1975.

Feifel, H.: "Death," in Farberow, N. (ed.), *Taboo Topics*, New York, Atherton Press, 1963.

Fleshman, R.: "The Health Care System of the Emergency Room," in Davis, M., et al. (eds.), *Nurses in Practice, A Perspective on Work Environments*, St. Louis, C. V. Mosby Co., 1975.

Gentry, W., and Haney, T.: "Emotional and Behavioral Reaction to Acute Myocardial Infarction," *Heart and Lung, The Journal of Critical Care*, 4(5):738–745, September–October 1975.

Glaser, B., and Strauss, A.: *Awareness of Dying*, Chicago, Aldine Publishing Co., 1965.

———, and ———: *A Time for Dying*, Chicago, Aldine Publishing Co., 1968.

Hackett, T., et al.: "The Coronary Care Unit, An Appraisal of Its Psychologic Hazards," *The New England Journal of Medicine*, 279(25):1365–1370, 1968.

Hamburg, D., et al.: "Adaptive Problems and Mechanisms in Severely Burned Patients," *Psychiatry, The Journal for the Study of Interpersonal Processes*, 16(1):1–20, February 1953.

Harper, B.: Keynote Address on *The Family and Death: A Social Work Symposium*, Foundation of Thanatology, Columbia-Presbyterian Medical Center, New York, April 12, 1975.

Holub, N., et al.: "Family Conferences as an Adjunct to Total Coronary Care," *Heart and Lung, The Journal of Critical Care*, 4(5):767–769, September–October 1975.

Jones, E.: "Who Supports the Nurse?" *Nursing Outlook*, 10(7):476–478, July 1962.

Kreiger, D.: "Therapeutic Touch," *American Journal of Nursing*, 75(5):784–787, May 1975.

Kübler-Ross, E.: "Crisis Management of Dying Persons and their Families," in Resnick, H. L. P., and Rubin, H. L. (eds.), *Emergency Psychiatric Care, The Management of Mental Health Crisis*, Bowie, Md., Charles Press Publishers, 1975.

Kuenzi, S., and Fenton, M.: "Crisis Intervention in Acute Care Areas," *American Journal of Nursing*, 75(5):830–834, May 1975.

Lazarus, R.: *Psychological Stress and the Coping Process*, New York, McGraw-Hill Book Co., 1966.

Lee, J.: "Emotional Reactions to Trauma," *The Nursing Clinics of North America*, 5(4):577–587, December 1970.

Lee, R., and Ball, P.: "Some Thoughts on the Psychology of the Coronary Care Unit," *American Journal of Nursing*, 75(9):1498–1501, September 1975.

McLachlan, E.: "Recognizing Pain," *American Journal of Nursing*, 74(3):496–497, March 1974.

Murphy, E.: "Intensive Nursing Care in a Respiratory Unit," *The Nursing Clinics of North America*, 3(3):423–436, September 1968.

Murray, R.: "Assessment of Psychologic Status in the Surgical ICU Patient," *The Nursing Clinics of North America*, 10(1):69–81, March 1975.

Obier, K., and Haywood, L.: "Enhancing Therapeutic Communication with Acutely Ill Patients," *Heart and Lung, The Journal of Critical Care*, 2(1):49–53, January–February, 1973.

Popoff, D., et al.: "What Are Your Feelings about Death and Dying, Part I," *Nursing 75*, 5(8):15–24, August 1975.

Quint, J.: "The Threat of Death: Some Consequences for Patients and Nurses," *Nursing Forum*, 8(3):287–300, 1969.

Roberts, S.: *Behavioral Concepts and the Critically Ill Patient*, Englewood Cliffs, N.J., Prentice-Hall, 1976.

Scalzi, C.: "Nursing Management of Behavioral Responses Following an Acute Myocardial Infarction," *Heart and Lung, The Journal of Critical Care*, 2(1):62–69, January–February, 1973.

Schichtmann, K.: "Adaptive Mechanisms in a Selected Group of Burn Patients," *ANA, Clinical Sessions—1968*, New York, Appleton-Century-Crofts, 1968.

Sobel, D.: "Personalization in the Coronary Care Unit," *American Journal of Nursing*, 69(7):1439–1442, July 1969.

Strauss, A.: "The Intensive Care Unit: Its Characteristics and Social Relationships," *The Nursing Clinics of North America*, 3(1):7–15, March 1968.

Taylor, C.: "The Hospital Patient's Social Dilemma," *American Journal of Nursing*, 65(10):96–99, October 1975.

Vreeland, R., and Ellis, G.: "Stresses on the Nurse in the Intensive Care Unit," *Journal of American Medical Association*, 206(2):332–334, April 1969.

Chapter 7

Care of the Chronically Dying

The most obvious difference between care of the acutely dying and that of the chronically dying is the trajectory, that is, the estimated time spent in dying. The chronically dying client may take months, sometimes years, and experience long plateaus characterized by varying degrees of wellness. The cancer client in remission, for instance, may be asymptomatic and feel very well, but on the other hand, the client with chronic renal failure who is on dialysis may never feel well. Both these clients have life-shortening chronic illnesses and may realistically be perceived as dying.

But to think of both these clients as indeed dying and therefore hopeless does them an injustice. It is still possible for them to function within a well model framework, making the most of remaining abilities and strengths by living each day to the fullest.

To the chronically dying client time is a double-edged sword. There is time to be with family, to continue to fulfill one's life goals, and to experience more living, but there is also time for anticipatory grief, diminished abilities, pain, acute exacerbations, and loneliness, all of which can precipitate crises. With acute exacerbations, the concepts discussed in regard to the acutely dying client are applicable, yet the underlying impact of continued chronic illness cannot be overlooked. In this manner, Chapters 6 and 7 are complementary.

After defining the chronically dying client, this chapter focuses on the application of the well model and crisis theory to the chronically dying client and includes the characteristics of chronic illness. The needs of the dying as detailed in Chapter 6 will also be applied to the chronically dying client. A special section on aging and the advantages and disadvantages of home versus institutional care will be presented. As with Chapter 6, this chapter focuses on nurses' problems in dealing with dying clients.

DEFINITION

Identifying when the dying process begins in chronic illness is a very difficult task. Dying may take place over months or even years. In retrospect, the beginning of the end may be seen as that point when the client noticeably began to deteriorate or when medication could no longer control the symptoms, but sometimes subtle changes can be overlooked in the lengthy process of a chronic illness.

This is not to say that chronic illness is to be equated with dying. Some chronic illnesses, although incapacitating and painful, are not life-shortening. No one ever died from the pain of arthritis, but it is a chronic illness with which one can associate loss and partial death: loss of health, loss of mobility, and loss of occupation.

Use of the Well Model

The well model, with its unitary focus, negative and positive potentials, and client advocacy, is an appropriate framework within which to view chronically ill and dying clients. They adapt holistically to the possibility of a shortened life span. Also, for some clients, such as those with cystic fibrosis or advanced cancer, the entire family life pattern may be severely modified to care for the client.

One does not have to look far to discover the negative potentials, or problems, in chronic illness. Increased physical disability, pain, family strain, and financial burden are some of its unpleasant realities. Medicine cannot cure it, and the physician can only hope to control the impact of the condition through periodic checkups. The nurse's role is limited to periodic guidance and to care during an acute exacerbation.

Notwithstanding negative potentials, clients with chronic illness often show remarkable ability to adapt and adjust. To do this, though, they must first acknowledge the problem, that is, accept the sick role and seek help. Temporary dependency is essential. The clients' resistance to viewing themselves as sick and now dependent is a significant factor in future adaptation and only increases stress.

The most common immediate response to threat of illness is denial and shock. Denial serves to temporarily minimize the threat, as a kind of preparation for future adjustment. Eventually there is recognition of the reality of the illness, seeking of treatment, and acceptance of temporary dependence. Simply stated, the change from healthy and independent proceeds to sick and dependent and, finally, to different and acceptable. The meaning of *different and acceptable* is aptly illustrated in the following vignette. A man was telling me about his 20-year-old retarded son. From the description, the son seemed quite severely impaired. The father said he was uneducable and had very poor speech. When I said that it must be very difficult for him to see his son so retarded, his reply was, "He is such a blessing." Yes his son was different, but also acceptable and lovable.

There are many ways clients and their families can be very inventive in the use of, in Strauss' words, "normalizing" tactics. These maneuvers, for the most part, are not taught by health care personnel but are developed by the client and the family, using the problem-solving process and trial and error. Normalizing tactics attempt to minimize or conceal symptoms, thereby assuming the maximum amount of wellness within the reality of the illness.

Nevertheless the task of living with the condition remains with the individual. In this situation one must be one's own long-term advocate and use one's abilities and strengths to maximize one's wellness and minimize one's illness. One must learn to monitor one's body, know the significance of signs and symptoms, and decide when it is necessary to see the doctor. To make life as normal as possible one learns to juggle regimes, medications, energy levels, finances, and appointments. One is the coordinator of one's own care. If one has several separate problems one takes the often fragmented and sometimes unrealistic advice from various sickness specialty care personnel and adapts it to oneself. Health care personnel can learn from this coordinator and advocate; he or she has first-hand knowledge of the reality of his or her illness. How the individual handles it needs to be included in the strength-oriented nursing record.

CRISIS THEORY

In contrast to the dramatic acutely dying setting, the chronically dying setting may seem an inappropriate place in which to apply crisis theory. Because of the slower pace of the illness, crisis situations may not even be identified until complete disorganization occurs. One kind of crisis occurs with realization of accumulated losses. The client who always hoped to return to work again may experience a crisis precipitated by the most recent loss, permanent unemployment. The advantage of the chronic illness, though, is the time available to try different adaptive maneuvers and to thus thwart potential crisis. The skillful and intuitive nurse may be able to anticipate a potential crisis situation and intervene before complete disorganization occurs.

A crisis for the chronically ill and dying client may occur when an exacerbation of or complications of the chronic illness require acute care. For example, increasing weakness in multiple sclerosis or leg amputation in the diabetic may bring on a crisis. The fact that people survive with a chronic illness gives credence to the tenacity and perseverance of the client and family members in adjusting. Some complications can be fatal, and this potential for death becomes a motivating factor in maintaining a close watch over symptoms.

The client and family members must organize for crisis management. Strauss discusses several ways in which this can be done. The client and family are taught to read the signs and symptoms and monitor the bodily changes that may precipitate a crisis, such as chest pain in the cardiac client. They also learn the measures to institute when a crisis occurs. An identification tag or card and telephone numbers tell strangers what to do and whom to call should an emergency arise. Some clients, in addition, carry equipment such as candy for the diabetic or extra colostomy bags to assist during an actual or potential crisis. In certain situations, such as hemophilia, entire environmental changes are necessary to keep an illness under control. Other illnesses require a high degree of structuring of daily life patterns because there are many time-consuming and complicated treatments.

A crisis may also occur with a breakdown in management of the illness and regime due to accident, ignorance, or a completely unexpected event such as a sudden new illness. Also, the client may relax vigilance as the time since the last crisis gets longer. In addition, if the people usually relied on to help are unavailable due to illness, separation, or abandonment, a medical crisis may occur.

For the most part families have developed measures for coping with strife, but sometimes novel or accumulated adversity can be crisis-precipitating. The family's value system and previous experience with crises determine how it views the event.

Social situations can also be crisis-precipitating. During the span of an illness, changes in relationships can occur. Role expectations, conceptions, performance, and acceptance change, and these changes often involve loss of status for clients. They become more dependent and less mobile. Individual members in a family may also become ill, die, move away, divorce, or abandon the household altogether. In short, all the problems confronting any family can also confront a family with a chronically ill member. The family as a unit is interdependent. When a problem develops with one member, a rebound effect occurs with all other members.

Not all the clients' social problems are the result of interactions of family members and friends. Some problems stem from a lack of any social relationship, progressive social isolation, and, in the extreme, social death. Examples of socially dead clients are those clients conscious but institutionalized who have completely lost the meaning of their existence.

When clients withdraw from social contacts because of increasing immobility or hearing or speech loss, they become isolated. The increasing demands on the clients of caring for their illness and increasing loss of energy diminish interest in social contacts. Bodily disfigurement may make either clients or friends and family withdraw. Changed interests and sphere of activity of clients, family, and friends may also diminish social contacts. Changing location, such as moving from home to institution or from one institution to another, may also increase isolation. Finally and most important is the difficulty experienced by friends and family as they watch the clients' progressive deterioration. Comforting words are hard to find and often sound hollow at this time, especially if the clients are expressing unpleasant emotions, depression and anger, or uncomfortable silences. Very few people can listen to a litany of complaints, and sometimes that is all chronically dying clients can offer. Consequently, family and friends abandon them.

The psychological crisis of the chronically dying client is related to losses, especially to those accumulating partial deaths that snowball into anticipatory grief. In contrast to the grief of bereavement, anticipatory grief escalates as the disease progresses and death draws ever nearer. Anticipatory grief is intrapsychically sadness and preoccupation with inevitable future losses. It especially is a real sense of the finality of life. Behaviorally, it is a form of patterned desocialization. This grief may last for a prolonged period of time, even until the moment of death.

Actual fear of death, according to Aldrich, is secondary to fear of losing loved ones when one dies. It is especially difficult for a strong, well-integrated personality to accept death with equanimity. The more resources a person has, the more the person has to lose. The conflict of separation is a formidable mountain to overcome.

In the dying process time is lost and with it a pervading sense of fulfillment. Goals and tasks may be left unresolved, and sometimes there is regret over misdeeds or unfinished tasks. Social contacts are important to the chronically dying client but may be diminishing. Therefore, the client experiences anticipatory grief, which is a long-lasting, lonely, sad, painful, and arduous task. Old age probably does not make it any easier. Even for the person with low social value to an onlooker, anticipatory grief can be a profound and bitter experience. Religious belief may also not provide significant comfort. There is no magic formula to minimize the impact of anticipatory grief. Often, too, it leaves the onlookers feeling helpless.

The client experiencing anticipatory grief may require crisis intervention for periodic severe episodes of disorganization and continued therapeutic intervention throughout the process. Responses to suffering depend on previous patterns of coping with stress, personality resources, and the amount of stress that must be faced in dying. Nurses who are willing to closely follow their clients may be able to anticipate a potentially critical period and therefore ease the strain.

NEEDS OF THE CHRONICALLY DYING CLIENT

Communication

The chronically dying setting has its own special communication problems. Clients still need to be able to interact with the social world. However, prolonged illness often imposes increasing restrictions. Clients see fewer and fewer people. The more ill they become, the more uncomfortable family and friends become. They may withdraw and completely abandon the clients emotionally.

Nurses can do much to maintain communication with chronically dying clients. First they should be aware of the avoidance behaviors they use toward clients and threatening situations, and they should make a conscious effort to eliminate these behaviors.

No matter how much has been written about therapeutic communication, there are only suggestions and guidelines to offer. Every person who has tried to be therapeutic when talking to a client will eventually realize, some more frequently than others, that the "right thing to say" sometimes escapes them and they can easily fall into meaningless talk because of embarrassment. Talking with the dying is filled with emotional land mines.

Communication cannot be isolated but must be viewed as part of the entire illness experience and accustomed pattern of communication. Talking serves many functions. Talking is a vehicle to establish contact with another person and to build a trusting relationship that helps relieve anxiety. Through talking one can plan, explain, and instruct. In addition, "talking is used to fill time. It can divert or amuse a patient, when he is so anxious that he must have time to structure his situation."* Talking and sharing, moreover, are essential to the anticipatory grief process, especially to accepting current and future losses and reviewing one's life. "An interim report from a study of loss and grief now in progress reveals a high incidence of guilt and regret among survivors who were unable to talk together and come to an acceptance shared with the dying family member."†

A willingness to listen is also an essential ingredient of productive communication. Listening conveys caring, shared feelings, and the beginning of a trusting relationship. Our ears hear; we listen with our whole selves. "Meaningful verbal communication is far more than an exchange of words. It is an exchange of understood meanings."‡ Of course, words can say only so much, but how they are said—the tone, mood, and attitude expressed—determine how they are received. Much can be said simply through shared silences, facial expressions, and body posture.

Another kind of nonverbal communication is touch. McCorkle found, in a study of 60 seriously ill clients, that touch can establish a quick rapport and a sense of caring. Kreiger, moreover, has demonstrated that *therapeutic touch* from a person trained in this technique is so powerful as to be able to raise the hemoglobin levels of clients.

The following are some guidelines for communicating with chronically dying clients:

*J. Craytor, "Talking with Persons Who Have Cancer," *American Journal of Nursing*, 69(4):746, April 1969.
    †Sister Z. Cotter, "On Not Getting Better," *Hospital Progress*, 63, March 1972.
    ‡Craytor, op. cit.

1   Allow the clients to set the pace. They will tell you when and how much information they want and can handle. If you are not sure whether a statement or question has some covert meaning, ask an open-ended question. This will help the clients become more specific and give you a better idea of what they are really saying or asking. It is essential, especially with dying clients, to find out very early in any relationship what they understand about their illness and what it means to them. That information can be obtained from the physician, from the chart, or directly from the client.

2   Never lie to a client. The client will lose trust in the care giver who lies. Usually clients who ask if they are dying want to be reassured that they will not be abandoned and will be kept comfortable, especially if they have a poor prognosis. Hope in the provision of comfort is essential. Comfort includes adequate pain relief.

3   Never ignore clients. The nurse who does not listen to the meaning of their words abandons clients emotionally. Physically, clients are abandoned when the nurse, for instance, avoids the clients' rooms and delays answering the call light. If a client wants to talk, pull up a chair and sit down. Listen. If you do not know what to say, say nothing. Even when conversation becomes extremely difficult, for instance, when a client is angry, depressed, silent, or crying, the presence of the nurse in the room silently says, "I accept your feelings."

A neglected aspect of communication is the intimacy and sexual needs of clients. Family and close friends can provide needed warmth and affection. Dying persons will feel abandoned if the persons with whom they meet their sexual needs do not find them sexually desirable. Unfortunately, a primitive fear of "catching" cancer, fear of hurting, or even revulsion may cause a spouse or lover, for instance, to move into another bedroom or even be afraid of embracing the dying client. Sexual intercourse is as appropriate in the dying as it is in the healthy, depending on the energy level and wishes of the dying person. Anticipatory guidance may minimize this problem, especially with cancer surgery.

Positive Body Image

Chronic illness and dying impose some frightening changes on the familiar healthy body. Outward appearance may change, normal functions may be diverted, whole parts may be lost. The person grieves over the lost body image before integrating the new body image with the old. In effect, the old self dies and a lengthy period of time elapses before the new self is born. Chapter 5 more fully discusses body image and its relation to illness.

In chronic illness, body-image changes may be permanent. Time is available to learn about these changes and to make adaptations in life patterns, including relationships of self to others. The chronically dying process also requires body-image change.

The following guidelines aim to restore and preserve positive body image:

   1   Do not force clients to do more than they can. Frequently, a nurse may think clients should be more self-sufficient than they really are at the moment. Body-image change and acceptance take time.
   2   The opposite situation can also occur. People may think the client with a disability in one area is completely incompetent; for example, the blind client is frequently thought of as much more helpless than is really so. Any and all measures to maximize independence will enhance body image.
   3   Because events happen slowly to the chronically ill and dying and the same problems exist for so long, creative approaches may be necessary for recalcitrant problems.
   4   Do not show revulsion at a changed body part, even though doing this is sometimes very difficult.
   5   Help make the client's life and appearance as normal as possible. Prostheses, for instance, serve as very effective camouflage for the mastectomy client.
   6   Part of building positive body image, and self-esteem in particular, is the social acceptability of the illness or disability. To enhance this feeling of acceptance, communication is crucial. Especially with an aphasic client, improvisation and perseverance are essential in gaining communication. For the client who is able to speak, listen as he or she sorts out feelings of anger and revulsion.
   7   Involve the family frequently in nursing care. They also need time to adapt to the family member's disability.

Physical Care

Most textbooks about psychological care ignore the physical needs of the client. For the dying, physical needs must be met in addition to psychological needs. Given all the disease possibilities, one cannot elaborate on all the kinds of physical care needed for the chronically dying client. The reader is advised to consult a medical-surgical nursing textbook for care of specific conditions, using the textbook only as a guide from which to individualize care.

   Another often overlooked determinant of physical care is the client's wishes. The physician and nurse must agree, within ethical boundaries, to provide the kind of care the client wishes.

   Specifically because dying clients have so little energy to meet their own needs, basic nursing measures to maintain comfort are essential. Sometimes this is all that can be done for the client. Measures such as frequent, gentle turning, easily digestible food, and prevention of impaction are basic but essential to client comfort. Always remember that the client's wishes must not be ignored. Finally, whatever else comfort care includes, it surely includes pain relief.

Control over One's Environment

To chronically dying clients any and all losses, such as loss of health, independence, social contacts, finances, and energy, portend lessened control over self and environment. Any control clients are able to maintain may of necessity be from a wheelchair or bed.

Notwithstanding the reality of the terminal illness and the client's increasing disability, the nurse can take positive steps to preserve thc client's control, self-esteem, dignity, and inherent strengths.

Some general guidelines for meeting this essential need are as follows:

1   Choices in care are necessary if clients are to be active participants in their care.

2   Adequate pain relief is essential if clients are to remain in control of their lives.

3   Environmental stimulation, for instance, social contacts and diversionary activities, relieve the sense of social isolation, worthlessness, and abandonment.

4   For the clients, home is probably the place most conducive to maintaining control over life and environment, but it is not always feasible for clients to remain at home. For those clients who choose to remain at home, support in terms of preparation for care and adequate ancillary services must be provided to cooperating family and client. The section in this chapter on home versus institutional care will be helpful in weighing the advantages and disadvantages of these choices.

Self-esteem

Self-esteem cannot be separated from the other needs of dying clients. Lack of attention to their nccds leads to a reduction in clients' self-esteem.

Simply stated, self-esteem is the overall fccling of worth a person has, which is closely linked to perception of a social self acceptable to the outside world. Self-esteem also plays an integral part in one's body image and individual value system. However, like health, self-esteem is impossible to break down into component parts without losing its essential quality.

According to Bibring, everyone aspires to be worthy (loved and appreciated), good (not aggressive or hateful), and strong (not dependent and helpless). Chronic illness and dying damage self-esteem by producing feelings of worthlessness, badness, and dependence.

Here are some suggestions for enhancing self-esteem:

1   Use the well model strength-oriented nursing record to clarify areas of strength and coping. Include those areas as part of nursing care; for instance, foster close family relationships by structuring the day to include more time for family visits.

2   Try to be increasingly sensitive to the effect your words and actions have on the client. The nurse may not be embarrassed by the client's constant diarrhea but the client might be, especially if he or she must use a bedpan in a room with other people.

3   Look for clues to low self-esteem. Derogatory remarks about self are

obvious, but covert clues, such as prolonged silences and slouched body posture, should not be overlooked.

4 As an advocate, the nurse should seek clients' opinions and give them choices in aspects of care. Genuine, not forced, compliments also are helpful.

Opportunity to Grieve for Themselves

The chronically ill grieve for many partial losses. Engle's model of adaptation to loss (see Chapter 5) is applicable to chronic illness also. The following is a brief summary of Crate's adaptation of Engle's model to chronic illness. She includes some suggestions for care.

1 *Disbelief* Clients have difficulty believing they have an illness. This serves to diminish the impact of the threat temporarily. The nurse should allow them to deny their illness by being a noncritical listener but should not actively support denial by, for instance, encouraging them not to seek medical assistance.

2 *Developing awareness* This stage may appear, for instance, as guilt over being sick, often expressed as anger. The nurse should encourage free expression of anger and guilt, but should not actively support it by, for example, blaming others for the client's affliction. Thus the client learns to accept care and depend on others, that is, to accept the sick role. Gradually the client will assume increasing responsibility.

3 *Reorganization* Body image, role expectations, and social identity change in relation to the disability. The family also needs time to adapt. The nurse listens nonjudgmentally to client and family in their newly evolving relationships.

4 *Resolution and identity change* At this point the clients have integrated their concept of self to include their illness or disability. They see themselves realistically as different from other people, limited in certain ways, but also functional. They move from well to sick to different.

This process is a continuous one, and for the terminally ill, each new loss may reactivate the cycle of grieving: denial, developing awareness, reorganization, and resolution.

Opportunity for a Life Review

The concept of the life review is usually associated with the elderly, but it is essential for all dying clients. The life review takes time and may occur periodically during the course of a lengthy dying period.

Briefly, the life review is spontaneous, unselective reminiscing about the past, especially about unresolved conflicts in the past. This free association allows for many unresolved conflicts to be looked at anew and, it is hoped, to be reconciled. If successful, the life review gives new meaning to one's life in preparation for death. It facilitates the "giving up" process of dying.

It is also a kind of mental scorecard on which is listed the attributes and deficiencies of a lifetime—accomplishments achieved and tasks left undone. The sum of these is the "worth" of one's life.

Guidelines for encouraging a life review are simple:

1   Listen.
2   Maintain confidentiality.

Relief from Pain

One of the most formidable challenges for a physician and nurse in the care of chronically dying clients is providing adequate pain relief. Chronic unremitting pain becomes a dehumanizing nightmare:

> Pain behavior in terminal conditions is strongly colored by the individual's feelings concerning impending death. Feelings of anxiety, for example, often lead to exaggerated pain complaint, and may actually intensify pain feelings as well. On the other hand, the expression of pain may disguise or camouflage feelings of depression occasioned by the real or the threatened loss of functions associated with the fatal illness.*

None of the other tasks of living while dying can be addressed when the client is overcome with pain. As pain takes control, the psychological repercussions increasingly are noticed. Health care personnel feel helpless and then angry as the client begs to receive medication before it is scheduled. They may even question the severity of the pain and call the client manipulative. For the most part, the United States is not known for its extraordinary record of pain relief for dying clients, that is, pain relief with the client remaining sentient. We need to be more flexible in terms of dosages, frequency, and kinds of drugs and should augment drugs with personal attention. More research into the efficacy of other pain-relief modalities, such as biofeedback and acupuncture, should be undertaken. As previously mentioned, St. Christopher's Hospice in London provides a flexible, regular schedule of pain medication liberally laced with heroin and alcohol.

Guidelines for pain relief are the same for the acutely dying client as given previously for the chronically dying client. They are as follows:

1   Give medication on time. Do not keep client waiting without a good explanation.
2   Monitor client's response to new medication.
3   Administer painful treatments when medication provides the most relief.
4   Encourage clients to use their own coping responses to pain.

*T. Gonda, "Pain and Addiction in Terminal Illness," in Schoenberg, B., et al. (eds.), *Loss and Grief: Psychological Management in Medical Practice*, New York, Columbia University Press, 1970, p. 264.

Spiritual Comfort

In contrast to the acutely dying, the chronically dying client has time to search for the meaning of life, an inherently spiritual task even for the person who claims to be agnostic or atheist. However, a strong religious faith does not necessarily make dying any easier.

Meeting the spiritual needs of clients is not solely the responsibility of the clergy. Nurses, in meeting the needs of clients, also minister to them. Spirituality is part of the whole person and cannot be compartmentalized. The most important guideline for nurses is to allow clients freedom to experience their own spirituality. In doing so nurses must not moralize or teach their own beliefs. Rather, they should listen carefully and purposefully.

The clergy also have an important role to play in the care of the dying. Visits from the hospital chaplain and the local clergy may be helpful. Certain religious rites and rituals are important to some clients just before and in the months preceding death.

Guidelines for the nurse to use in allowing the client time for spiritual comfort are the same as those for the acutely dying:

1 Listen carefully to the client's expression of beliefs.
2 Provide time for the client to be alone and reflect.
3 Encourage visits by the clergy if the client so desires.

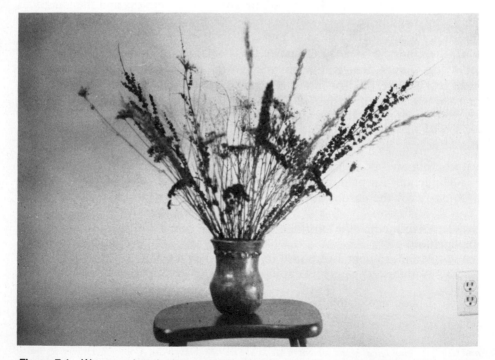

Figure 7-1 We appreciate the beauty of old, dried flowers—why not the beauty of old people?

AGING
Well Model

Eighty-six percent of the elderly have at least one chronic illness. For this group of people the earlier part of this chapter is applicable in addition to the following developmental aspects of dying. However, aging by itself must not be considered synonymous with illness, senility, or incompetence. The remaining 14 percent of the elderly are, in the usual sense of the word, healthy. Even a portion of the 86 percent with chronic illnesses are functionally healthy, and all have some strengths. If, therefore, the focus of care were on capability and not on disability, iatrogenic illness and dependency would be less of a problem.

The well model is an appropriate framework for care of the elderly. There are many positive potentials to be assessed and utilized. Adaptability in the older person (and in the younger person also) depends on pre-existent personality traits, sense of social worth, and functional ability. Physical health, in addition, is a major determinant of adaptability. Today's elderly people have weathered many difficulties and hardships in the past. Many elderly persons remain creative and curious throughout their entire lifetimes. (See Figures 7-1 and 7-2.) They are willing to share their accumulated experience, wisdom, and insight, which Butler calls the "elder" function:

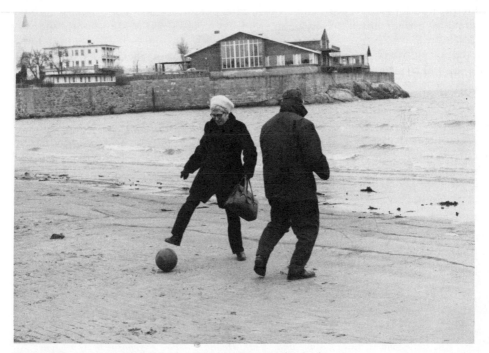

Figure 7-2   Youth is a state of mind that can rule an aging body.

Insight requires not only an inner sense of one's self and motivation, but also an inner knowledge of human life cycle—a realization of life and how it changes . . . includes a willingness and ability to substitute available satisfaction for losses incurred.*

Because of these positive potentials, the elderly are ready and able to be their own health care advocates. Aging does have its negative potentials, though. The next section, on crisis theory and aging, describes many of these possibilities.

Recent research has not clearly identified those changes that are exclusively related to aging and those that are illness-related. Intelligence, for the most part, remains unchanged with aging. Some physical characteristics of aging include gray hair, wrinkled skin, sagging body posture, and diminished hearing and eyesight. Along with these changes there is a concomitant body-image change.

The elderly person has new roles to fulfill and tasks to accomplish in addition to those continued from earlier years. Retirement brings new leisure time, decreased income, modifications in life-style, and sometimes the need for supplemental income, changes that utilize previous and sometimes new interests and abilities. Outside interests may include social, civic, and political responsibility. Modifications in living may include finding new housing appropriate to health and economic status. Maximizing health requires adequate health and sickness care from health care personnel and good health habits, such as proper nutrition, hygiene, and exercise. Relationships with spouse, other family members, and old and new friends help retain a sense of meaning to life. The elderly person must come to terms with illness and death of a spouse, family member, friends, and self. Part of the task of coming to terms with death is developing a personal philosophy of living.

Crisis Theory

Even healthy elderly people have problems, and some of these, depending on current ability to solve problems, may reach crisis proportions. A crisis, for example, can occur with the perception of loss. The constant losses of aging may produce a kind of chronic grief. When a period of disequilibrium ensues, the elderly sometimes hesitate to seek help because they fear loss of autonomy by inappropriate institutionalization.

Notwithstanding previous strengths and adaptiveness, aging cannot be hidden with hair dye and youthful clothes. Implications of aging can be crisis-producing. Loss of youth, that highly prized American value, and integration of the idea of oneself as old or elderly is a major adjustment for the older person.

In terms of the losses caused by *chronic illness*, many kinds of temporary

*R. Butler and M. Lewis, *Aging and Mental Health, Positive Psychosocial Approaches*, St. Louis: C. V. Mosby Co., 1973, p. 18.

crises can occur. The recently *bereaved and widowed* experience increased medical and psychiatric morbidity and mortality. *Sexual problems* of the married can often follow recent surgery, illness, or bereavement. Following the strict sexual customs of their youth, the unmarried frequently find extramarital sex unacceptable. *Retirement*, a maturational crisis, may bring on a sense of uselessness and boredom. With retirement comes *decreased income*, a major pervasive problem: one out of every four elderly lives below the poverty line. *Sensory loss* can reduce reality testing and can lead to marked suspiciousness and even paranoia, depression, and social isolation.

A crisis resulting from decreased income, chronic illness, sensory loss, depression, and lack of information is the inability to maintain *nutritional status*. Some old people literally starve to death. *Immobilization*, resulting from a chronic illness or sensory loss or even loss of a driver's license, is also a crisis-precipitating event for the elderly. In cities, the aged fear *robberies and muggings*. When these occur a crisis ensues.

Another example of a potential crisis situation is the constant, recurrent, or nagging pain that often accompanies the aged person without chronic illness. This pain increases the person's sense of vulnerability and decreases the sense of control over one's body. Hospitalization is often viewed by the elderly as a portent of death. The person may also feel isolated, bored, and hopeless if confined to or in institutions. *Surgery*, as with any physical stress, can cause serious disorientation, pain, fright, and especially the fear of death. *Falls* and *fractures* are a frequent occurrence for the elderly. Sometimes they lie on the floor for hours or days before help arrives. Upon awakening in the morning some elderly experience "little strokes," which include temporary periods of confusion, disorientation, and garbled speech. They are a frightening occurrence for the elderly. Moreover, many elderly take many kinds of medication, the inadvertent misuse of which can cause a crisis. *Fire* is always a potential threat to those living in institutions or rundown hotels. When fire does occur the loss may include personal belongings and friends and may cause injury and confusion.

Relocation of the elderly also may be a cause of crisis. Some persons tolerate change of rooms or homes poorly, becoming disoriented and frightened. Involuntary relocation may not just increase loneliness and social isolation, but may also increase morbidity and mortality. An especially sad and difficult problem is the newly institutionalized elderly person. He or she may feel family rejection and loss of home and possessions, privacy and independence, self-identity, self-esteem, and individuality. Moreover the elderly person may feel frustrated, insecure, and anxious in the new surroundings.

Finally, *death of self*, a potential maturational crisis, must be contemplated by the elderly. Not all elderly persons fear death, although many fear that they will die alone. Reactions to death are closely related to a sense of fulfillment and to the significance of one's contribution to others.

Each person knows what a good, appropriate personal death would be. The elderly know what they want in terms of how they live and how they die, and they should be asked. An instance arose of a woman facing death who invited three undertakers for lunch so that she could determine which one had the most to offer her. One undertaker declined the invitation because "he had never interviewed the deceased before." The woman made her choice of undertaker as well as selecting the priest to celebrate her funeral mass (because he had the best singing voice) and the biblical texts to be read at the services.

With all the aforementioned potential crisis situations, the elderly continue to live because of their strengths and adaptability. If their usual problem-solving measures become ineffective, however, this can lead to increased feelings of fear and vulnerability. Then the crisis-intervention model is an effective approach in restoring equilibrium and may even be a vehicle for improving previous well-being. A crisis is an opportunity to grow even for the elderly.

Dying

The elderly have reached that last stage of life, in which, as Erikson observes, one must come to terms with death. Feifel feels that "adaptation of the older person to dying and death, for example, may well be a crucial aspect of the aging process."* In addition, Weisman and Hackett's concept of appropriate death is also applicable; appropriate death may be different for each person.

A new concept, *life cycle theory*, sheds some light on how a person views death with equanimity. This theory is an embryonic attempt to describe the normative and modal changes inherent in the rhythm of life. An important part of the adaptation in any life phase is a developing sense of the life cycle: its rhythm, variability, and relation to sense of self. Possibly because of the older person's sense of life's rhythm and the past, the sense of time is somewhat different from that of a younger person. A younger person often cannot conceive of the future not existing, but for the older person the future is today. He or she has a sense of presence and immediacy, a sense of living for the moment. Age, for the elderly, is looked upon not as distance from the beginning but as nearness to the end.

The meaning of death for the elderly reflects their sense of consummation or fulfillment in life, and the life review can help them identify that sense of accomplishment. Their attitudes toward death depend upon many factors: chronological age, distance from death, physical and mental health, and influence of varying frames of references, such as religion, community attitudes, family and personal experience with death, attitudes of people in the immediate environment, psychological maturity and integrity, and past experiences in adjusting to crisis and change.

To many, death is much more than a biological event. Although there are conflicting viewpoints, most elderly fear death less than they fear prolonged illness; dependency; pain; rejection; isolation; and loss of social role, self-determination, and dignity.

*H. Feifel, "Attitudes toward Death in Some Normal and Mentally Ill Populations," in Feifel, H. (ed.), *The Meaning of Death*, New York: McGraw-Hill Book Co., 1959, p. 128.

HOME VERSUS INSTITUTIONAL CARE

The great majority of clients die in hospitals or nursing homes ostensibly because better care is available there than at home. Health care workers are paid to provide skilled comfort care and, in particular, perform treatments and give medications.

For client and kin, hospitalization relieves them of much of the responsibility of care. Sometimes the emotional drain of 24-hour care for a dying family member cannot be tolerated. Moreover, the care giver at home may not be strong enough to do the necessary lifting and other tasks. Perhaps everyone in the family works and the ill member cannot be left alone. The saddest situation occurs, of course, when there are no family members or friends available at any time.

The trade-off inherent in skilled comfort care is its attendant coldness. Hospital and nursing home routine continues around dying clients, and they must adjust even though their sense of time is different from the hospital's. Institutionalized dying clients relinquish their rights, especially personal privacy, and abrogate their responsibilities to sickness care workers.

Hospitals are designed for the living. Glaser and Strauss, Sudnow and Mendelson are but a few of the people describing the plight of the dying in institutions: avoided and ignored by doctors and nurses who, behind their professional demeanor, feel helpless, powerless, and angry.

Not all institutional care is cold. In the United States the hospice movement, modeled on St. Christopher's in London, is only beginning. Throughout the country hospices are being planned and built to provide comfort and supportive care without extraordinary measures. Clients are given more choices in their care. Moreover, a strong emphasis is placed on maintaining family ties.

Some clients elect to die at home, and family members agree to provide the necessary care. Care at home is cheaper than hospitalization, especially in prolonged illness. Clients, moreover, retain more control over their own care and environment. Too, home care may be the final act of love and responsibility for the dying family member.

Home care of the dying, therefore, must be viewed within a family framework. The nurse must provide the family with sufficient information and support to (1) care for the dying member and (2) help maintain as normal a pattern of family functioning as possible. Specifically, the nurse must prepare the family for the emotional ramifications of dying and for what to expect as death draws near. Ancillary personnel can provide essential support in keeping clients at home.

Sometimes family members think they have more stamina than they actually have. Therefore, the option of clients' returning to the hospital should be presented in a fashion that will minimize feelings of guilt and defeat.

There can also be obstacles to teaching family members the appropriate care. Some people, for one reason or another, have difficulty learning the tasks, and some are offended by aspects of care, such as odors. Then there are families who insist upon giving care their way.

For home care of the dying to have maximum therapeutic effect, good interpersonal relationships within the family are a must. Not every family has the ideal warm, supportive relationships, and the dying process may exacerbate long-standing problems.

In addition, family members, especially the primary care giver, frequently have unmet needs during this time. Most time and energy must be spent on the ill member, leaving little or no time for emotional or diversional outlets for care givers. A periodic respite from 24-hour responsibility is essential if the care giver is to remain healthy. Moreover, the primary care giver needs to know that he or she is not alone but has the support of family members and health care personnel. Finally, emergency telephone numbers should be readily available.

Cancer Care, Inc., in New York is an organization providing free comprehensive care to advanced cancer clients and their families. Services include counseling to meet crises and support of the strengths of clients and families. The organization tries to help families keep clients home as long as possible.

NURSES' REACTIONS

Problems with the Client and the Setting

Just as the nurse in the acute care setting has a myriad of pressures inhibiting good psychological care, so the nurse caring for the chronically dying also has conflicts. The sense of omnipotence, the working-toward-cure orientation, and the need to feel competent all exist in the chronic setting.

Nurses care for chronically dying clients in rehabilitation or chronic disease hospitals, nursing homes, or the medical-surgical areas of acute care hospitals. Public health and visiting nurses, in addition, are frequently in contact with the chronically dying in their homes. Nurses in out-patient departments and places such as kidney dialysis centers also care for chronically dying clients.

The chronic setting has built-in dangers for nurses, and these dangers are escalated by the time factor. There is more time to get to know the client, more time to try to cure, more time to grieve, and more time to experience a client's social loss:

> He cannot be avoided or forgotten all the time, and nurses tend to become involved simply as a consequence of long-term contact with him and his family. . . . They expect to see the patient each day as part of coming to work. They become good friends with him, expecting regular exchanges with him and enjoying the daily job of making him comfortable. If he is alternately going home and returning to the ward as his condition varies, he is welcomed as an old friend each time he returns. After a time, some nurses may develop a ''never will die'' expectation for the patient, which weakens their emotional defenses so that when he finally dies, loss of composure is more likely.*

*B. Glaser and A. Strauss, *Awareness of Dying*, Chicago, Aldine Publishing Co., 1965, p. 239.

Clients who have repeated admissions have diseases characterized by re-missions and exacerbations. They are the kind of people for whom the "never will die" attitude can develop, for example, those with cancer, multiple scle-rosis, and cirrhosis of the liver.

In order for nurses to experience interpersonal conflict and grief in the dying process they must first recognize the dying process in their clients. In the American culture, the physician is the only one who can legitimately define a client as dying, but nurses assess clues from clients' appearance, behavior, and chart, and physician's direct and indirect information. Intuition also plays a part in this assessment. Once aware of the dying process nurses tailor their involvement according to a perceived expected dying trajectory: quick or slow. These predictions of the trajectory and nurses' knowledge of clients' awareness of their terminality are the basis for nurses' varying degrees of involvement and composure. Often the perceived dying trajectory is not synchronized with the actual dying process; therefore, constant attention must be paid to adjusting strategies for and care of the client.

For the nurse, the client, and sometimes the family, a crisis can be created by the termination of a significant relationship. The most dramatic and most poignant is the death of a client. Kelly states that because we intuitively value close relationships, we feel it is constructive to experience the anguish of terminating a relationship. The longer the significant relationship, the more intense the feeling. The relationship with a client becomes significant when much time, effort, and energy are expended in giving lifesaving or comfort care or in just sharing the remissions and exacerbations of a chronic illness. "Loss is simultaneously a real event and perception by which the individual endows the event with personal or symbolic meaning. . . . Symbolic or anticipated loss, just as actual loss, may produce intense and sometimes pathologic reactions."*

Kelly suggests several mechanisms nurses use to minimize loss and avoid resolving feelings: (1) substituting someone else for the lost relationship, (2) imagining that the person still exists, (3) withdrawing from involvement, (4) identifying with the lost person by taking on that person's mannerisms, clothing, and interests, (5) denying and repressing the significance of the relationship, and (6) rationalizing that the relationship was not important anyway. Ration-alizing is another form of denying.

Other ways nurses cope with threatened loss are by using social distancing behaviors, attitudes, and words. Some were mentioned in the chapter on the acutely dying client. Glaser and Strauss detail many such maneuvers, for ex-ample, directing conversation away from potentially threatening topics. Blatant avoidance is used when other techniques are too threatening. A nurse can avoid the client by delaying answering the call bell, by forgetting the client, or by directly asking someone else to care for the client. It would behoove each nurse

*D. Peretz, "Development, Object-Relationships, and Loss," in Schoenberg, B., et al. (eds.), *Loss and Grief, Psychological Management in Medical Practice*, New York, Columbia University Press, 1970, p. 6.

to make a list of how many times a day and in what ways contact with a dying client has been successfully avoided.

Still another way of evading the stress of dying clients is to choose an area of work with a low mortality rate, such as obstetrics or psychiatry. Moving frequently from job to job or ward to ward also minimizes involvement.

Just as the acute care setting must build in emotional supports for the nurse, so, also, must the chronic care setting. The need in the chronic setting may be less dramatic and obvious because of the slower pace of the dying trajectory, but the degree of personal loss is greater because the client is known for a long time. Also, the nurse in the chronic setting may be less prepared for death than colleagues in the acute setting because dying happens less frequently.

Possible Solutions

Many of the measures mentioned in the chapter on the acutely dying client could be implemented in the chronic setting to ensure sufficient time to grieve. First, acknowledgment by peers and the administration of the nurse's need to grieve would serve two purposes. It would legitimize that need for the nurse and might even hasten the time when psychosocial care is actually an account-able part of nursing care. Second, sufficient time off is essential. Third, informal group meetings with a consultant to talk over feelings would be helpful. In the chronic setting, oncology and geriatric nurses are especially vulnerable to grief. There is much long-term contact with their clients.

In addition to working through staff grief, identifying potentially dying clients and developing possible strategies for their care are also necessary. In many instances, clients in the chronic setting are not identified as dying if they are weeks and sometimes days from dying. Obviously, to care for dying clients adequately one must first identify them as dying and then plan care. The use of the psychological autopsy can be helpful as a review in retrospect. Under-standing gained from the use of the psychological autopsy will help the nurse become more sensitive about recognizing when this phase begins with future clients.

SUMMARY

The characteristics, problems, and definition of the chronically dying client are, in many respects, quite different from those of the acutely dying client. Time runs slowly for the chronically dying. By definition the chronically dying patient expires over a period of months and years, with probably no clear signal point or dividing line when the terminal period begins. A prolonged dying trajectory can produce many problems that the acutely dying trajectory does not. Clients' responses to suffering depend upon their previous patterns of coping with stress, their personality resources, and amount of stress they must face in dying.

The characteristics of chronic illness and dying are discussed in a broad interactional framework. Well model concepts are applicable. Negative potentials for chronically dying clients may include increased physical disability, pain, anticipatory grief, financial burden, and family strain. At many points any of these problems can produce a crisis. The alert nurse may be able to intervene to prevent a crisis from occurring or to defuse it when it happens. Some positive potentials clients may be using are "normalizing" tactics, family support, and the ability to accept the sick role and, therefore, accept help. They may also be able to monitor bodily needs, changes, and energy levels. Clients must be their own advocates, with periodic intervention by health care personnel.

The needs of the chronically dying include communication, positive body image, self-esteem, life review, grief, pain relief, physical care, control over environment, and spiritual comfort. Suggestions for the nurse's role in meeting these needs are detailed. Essentially, the nurse should approach the client with openness, truthfulness, support, acceptance (especially of physical changes), care choices, pain relief, and a listening technique that will ferret out the client's underlying meanings. The nurse must also be flexible, have realistic expectations of the client, try to establish a sense of normalcy, and encourage family involvement.

Because 86 percent of the elderly have at least one chronic illness, and the elderly are at the end of their lives, aging is discussed in terms of the well model, crisis theory, and dying. The elderly have many positive potentials with which to cope with daily living; they have the adaptability to have weathered many hardships; many are in relatively good health. Ultimately adaptability for the elderly depends upon preexistent personality traits, sense of social worth, and functional ability. Many elderly persons are able to be their own advocates. However, the elderly have many losses with which to cope, and these losses can be crisis-precipitating. Some of these problems the elderly must deal with are chronic illness, bereavement and widowhood, sexual problems, retirement, decreased income, sensory loss, diminished nutritional status, immobilization, criminal assaults, pain, hospitalization, surgery, falls and fractures, "little strokes," inadvertent misuse of medications, fire, relocation, and death of self. In relation to dying, many elderly persons do not fear it less than they fear the above mentioned losses. The aged person's attitudes toward death depend upon chronological age, distance from death, physical and mental health, and influence of varying frames of reference, such as religion, community attitudes, family and personal experience with death, attitudes of persons in the immediate environment, psychological maturity and integrity, and past experiences in adjusting to crisis and change.

The majority of chronically dying clients die in hospitals or nursing homes. Some advantages to dying in an institution are the availability of skilled personnel and the removal of 24-hour care responsibility from the family, but the client in the hospital or nursing home must tolerate the cold and impersonal environment, relinquish some rights, especially the right to personal privacy, and abrogate responsibility to sickness care workers. To alleviate this problem the hospice movement in the United States, patterned after St. Christopher's Hospice in London, has burgeoned in recent years.

Some clients elect to die at home. The nurse is in a crucial position to support the client and family through the process. Family teaching must include not only client's treatments and medications, but also the family's need to remain healthy and maintain as normal a family life as possible.

Finally, nurses in the chronically dying setting are at risk because they grieve for their dying clients. The longer they know the clients the more they grieve. Frequently nurses use avoidance behaviors and mental mechanisms to minimize threat of loss. Some of the emotional supports mentioned in Chapter 6 on acutely dying, are also applicable to chronically dying; examples are sufficient time off and informal group meetings.

The final chapter will discuss curriculum strategies and guidelines for teaching nursing students about dying.

QUESTIONS FOR REFLECTION AND DISCUSSION

7-1 List all clients on your unit who have potentially life-shortening chronic illnesses. Is this unit a general medical-surgical unit of an acute care hospital or a chronic disease hospital? Or is this another kind of institution?
   a Have any clients been identified as dying? If yes, has care changed since that identification? In what ways has care changed?
   b Are clients aware of their terminality?
7-2 In terms of awareness, what kinds of conversations with dying clients are (a) easiest and (b) most difficult for you?
7-3 What is social loss? How does it affect nursing care?
7-4 Choose a client with a potentially life-shortening chronic illness (for example, cirrhosis of liver). How long has he or she had this condition?
   a Identify the major medical, social, and psychological stresses in the client's life at present.
   b Identify the ways the person copes with them.
   c Can you identify any recent losses in the client's life? If so, how has adaptation to these losses occurred? Is he or she grieving in anticipation of future losses?
   d When not hospitalized, what outside resources (pharmacy, visiting nurses) does the client use?
   e What are his or her activities of daily living in the hospital? At home? Is assistance required with any of these activities?
   f Does he or she have any recreational or diversionary activities?
   g What normalizing tactics are used?
   h What major fears does this client express?
   i What are this client's developmental tasks? How does the client meet them while in the hospital? How does the client meet them outside the hospital?
   j In what ways does the family help or hinder the client's progress?
   k What kinds of diversionary activity does the major family care giver still have? What are this person's current eating and sleeping patterns?
   l How is normalcy maintained within the family unit when the chronically dying member is at home?

     m Does this client also have an acute illness now? If so, how are acute and chronic needs similar and/or different?

     n Identify behavior that demonstrates changes in independence and dependence. Self-image and body image. Role.

     o What are the discharge plans for this client? Has the client been consulted? What extra supports might the client need?

7-5 Compare and differentiate the needs, strengths, and problems of two clients with the same diagnosis.

7-6 Choose an elderly client.

     a Answer all questions in no. 4 in relation to this client.

     b What extra stresses and adaptations are necessary because of age?

7-7 Ask five colleagues their feelings about taking care of older clients and dying clients.

7-8 How open or visible is death or dying in the chronic care setting? How is visibility controlled? Where are dying clients located spatially or physically?

7-9 In terms of division of labor, who manages the pre- and postdeath tasks in the hospital?

BIBLIOGRAPHY

Aguilera, D., and Messick, J.: *Crisis Intervention, Theory and Methodology*, St. Louis, C. V. Mosby Co., 1974.

Aldrich, C.: "The Dying Patient's Grief," *Journal of American Medical Association*, **184**(5):329–331, May 4, 1963.

————: "Some Dynamics of Anticipatory Grief," in Schoenberg, B., et al. (eds.), *Anticipatory Grief*, New York, Columbia University Press, 1974.

Bambino, C.: "Surveillance in Long-Term Illness," in Davis, M., et al. (eds.), *Nurses in Practice, A Perspective on Work Environments*, St. Louis, C. V. Mosby Co., 1975.

Benoleil, J.: "Anticipatory Grief in Physicians and Nurses," in Schoenberg, B., et al. (eds.), *Anticipatory Grief*, New York, Columbia University Press, 1974.

————: "Talking with Patients about Death," *Nursing Forum*, **9**(3):254–269, 1970.

Bibring, E.: "The Mechanisms of Depression," in Greenacre, P. (ed.), *Affective Disorders*, New York, International Universities Press, 1953.

Blackwell, B.: "Stigma," in Carlson, C. (ed.), *Behavioral Concepts in Nursing Intervention*, Philadelphia, J. B. Lippincott Co., 1970.

Burnside, I.: *Nursing and the Aged*, New York, McGraw-Hill Book Co., 1976.

Butler, R., and Lewis, M.: *Dying and Mental Health, Positive Psychosocial Approaches*, St. Louis, C. V. Mosby Co., 1973.

Carpentier, J., and Wylie, C.: "Aging, Dying and Denying," *Public Health Reports*, **89**(5):403–407, September–October 1974.

Cotter, Sister Z.: "On Not Getting Better," *Hospital Progress*, 60–63, March 1972.

Crate, M.: "Nursing Functions in Adaptation to Chronic Illness," *American Journal of Nursing*, **65**(10):72–76, October 1965.

Craven, J., and Wald, F.: "Hospice Care for Dying Patients," *American Journal of Nursing*, **75**(10):1816–1822, October 1975.

Craytor, J.: "Talking with Persons Who Have Cancer," *American Journal of Nursing*, **69**(4):744–748, April 1969.

Davis, M.: "The Public Health Nurse: Some Aspects of Work," in Davis, M., et al.

(eds.), *Nurses in Practice, A Perspective on Work Environments*, St. Louis, C. V. Mosby Co., 1975.

Diers, D., et al: "The Effect of Nursing Interaction on Patients in Pain," *Nursing Research*, **21**(5):419–428, September–October 1972.

Erikson, E.: *Childhood and Society*, 2d ed., New York, W. W. Norton and Co., 1963.

Feifel, H.: "Attitudes toward Death in Some Normal and Mentally Ill Populations," in Feifel, H. (ed.), *The Meaning of Death*, New York, McGraw-Hill Book Co., 1959.

————: "Older Persons Look at Death," *Geriatrics*, 127–130, March 1956.

Feldman, D.: "Chronic Disabling Illness: A Holistic View," *Journal of Chronic Disease*, **27**:287–291, 1974.

Glaser, B., and Strauss, A.: "Pain," in Davis, M., et al. (eds.), *Nurses in Practice: A Perspective on Work Environments*, St. Louis, C. V. Mosby Co., 1975.

Gonda, T.: "Pain and Addiction in Terminal Illness," in Schoenberg, B., et al. (eds.), *Loss and Grief: Psychological Management in Medical Practice*, New York, Columbia University Press, 1970.

Hill, R.: "Generic Features of Families Under Stress," in Parad, H. (ed.), *Crisis Intervention: Selected Readings*, New York, Family Service Association of America, 1965.

Jeffers, F., and Verwoerdt, A.: "How the Old Face Death," in Bussee, E., and Pheiffer, E. (eds.), *Behavior and Adaptation in Late Life*, Boston, Mass., Little, Brown and Co., 1969.

Jennings, M., et al.: "Physiologic Functioning in the Elderly," *The Nursing Clinics of North America*, **7**(2):237–252, June 1972.

Kelly, H.: "The Sense of an Ending," *American Journal of Nursing*, **69**(11):2378–2381, November 1969.

Kreiger, D.: "Therapeutic Touch," *American Journal of Nursing*, **75**(5):784–787, May 1975.

Kutscher, A.: "Psychopharmacological and Analgesic Agents in Care of the Dying Patient: For What End?" *Journal of Thanatology*, **2**(1–2):610–614, Winter–Spring 1972.

Lange, S.: "Shame," in Carlson, C. (ed.), *Behavioral Concepts in Nursing Intervention*, Philadelphia, J. B. Lippincott Co., 1970.

Leonard, B.: "Body Image in Chronic Illness," *The Nursing Clinics of North America*, **7**(4):687–695, December 1972.

Levin, J., and Kahana, R. (eds.), *Psychodynamic Studies on Aging: Creativity, Reminiscing and Dying*, New York, International Universities Press, 1969.

McCorkle, R.: "Effects of Touch on Seriously Ill Patients," *Nursing Research*, **23**(2):125–132, March–April 1974.

Mendelson, M.: *Tender Loving Greed*, New York, Alfred A. Knopf, 1974.

Murray, R., and Zentner, J.: *Nursing Assessment and Health Promotion through the Life Span*, Englewood Cliffs, N.J., Prentice-Hall, 1975.

Pattison, E.: "Psychosocial and Religious Aspects of Medical Ethics," in William, R. (ed.), *To Live and to Die: When, Why, How*, New York, Springer-Verlag, 1973.

Peretz, D.: "Development, Object-Relationships, and Loss," in Schoenberg, B., et al. (eds.), *Loss and Grief: Psychological Management in Medical Practice*, New York, Columbia University Press, 1970.

Reeves, R.: "The Hospital Chaplain Looks at Grief," in Schoenberg, B., et al. (eds.), *Loss and Grief: Psychological Management in Medical Practice*, New York, Columbia University Press, 1970.

Schoenberg, B., and Senescu, R.: "The Patient's Reaction to Fatal Illness," in Schoen-
    berg, B., et al. (eds.), *Loss and Grief: Psychological Management in Medical
    Practice*, New York, Columbia University Press, 1970.
Strauss, A.: *Chronic Illness and the Quality of Life*, St. Louis, C. V. Mosby Co., 1975.
————, and Glaser, B.: *A Time for Dying*, Chicago, Aldine Publishing Co., 1968.
Sudnow, D.: *Passing On: The Social Organization of Dying*, Englewood Cliffs, N.J.,
    Prentice-Hall, 1967.
Verwoerdt, A., and Wilson, R.: "Communication with the Fatally Ill, Tacit or Explicit,"
    American Journal of Nursing, **57**(11):2307–2309, November 1967.
Vincent, P.: "The Sick Role in Patient Care," *American Journal of Nursing*,
    75(7):1172–1173, July 1975.
Weisenberg, M. (ed.), *Pain, Clinical and Experimental Perspectives*, St. Louis, C. V.
    Mosby Co., 1975.
Weisman, A.: *The Realization of Death, A Guide for the Psychological Autopsy*, New
    York, Jason Aronson, 1974.
————, and Hackett, T.: "Predilection to Death, Death and Dying as a Psychiatric
    Problem," *Psychosomatic Medicine*, **23**(3):232–255, 1961.

Chapter 8

Curriculum Guidelines

This final chapter proposes guidelines for teaching care of the dying client to nursing students and nurses. Death and dying must be integrated with life's natural continuum. The many hours spent in maternal and child health, studying the birth process, growth, and development, must be complemented by studying the dying process. In fact, concepts inherent in the study of the dying process can be applied throughout the life span. Loss occurs, for example, not only in dying but also when a newborn loses the mother's womb, an adolescent loses a friend, or an adult loses a job. All these losses are partial deaths.

Nurses in every clinical setting inevitably encounter the dying process in both their clients and themselves. In obstetrics and psychiatry, deaths are infrequent but usually very traumatic. Even the nurse in the health maintenance organization cares for both chronically dying and recently bereaved clients.

Understanding the dying process and providing therapeutic care should not be left to periodic visits of a consulting specialist, even if he or she can see the person every day. It is especially important for the 24-hours-a-day, every-day care givers to be able to approach the dying client with understanding that gives meaning to living while dying. Along with understanding, consistent, constant, and compassionate care makes the dying process easier and less traumatic.

The concepts presented in this book are basic and can be taught under a variety of circumstances, appropriately modified for different levels of nursing schools and in-service education for staff nurses and faculty. Since nurses' aides are often the direct care givers, their education on dying should not be neglected. A nurse does not need an advanced degree to give comprehensive care to a dying client.

INTEGRATED VERSUS SEPARATE COURSE

Each institution will decide how death and dying best fits into its curriculum. Death education courses have been taught under the auspices of philosophy, theology, anthropology, psychology, sociology, health education, medicine, nursing departments, and even all levels of elementary and secondary schools. The concepts of death and dying can be taught in an integrated or a separate course. There are advantages and disadvantages to both approaches.

Integrated Course

Advantages   Since death and dying is experienced by the student, beginning usually in an anatomical dissection class, it is appropriate to present these concepts throughout the curriculum. This approach facilitates gradual maturation of personal feelings and knowledge. The student has more time to reflect on specific issues, to clarify values, and to solve complex issues and situations. In addition, the usefulness of specific concepts such as the well model, loss, body image, and pain may be expanded beyond the obviously dying client to various other settings and life experiences.

Disadvantages   The quality of instruction and guidance may vary greatly with the interest and ability of various teachers. This problem can be remedied by provision for faculty in-service education and use of one consultant to teach the death-related content, but the quality of concomitant clinical experience cannot be assured without further faculty improvements.

Separate Course

Advantages   One person teaching the separate course, using appropriate resource people, would provide more uniform and controlled instruction. This person's extensive knowledge of the field of thanatology would provide a more complete in-depth program.

Disadvantages   It is difficult to decide whether a separate course should be placed at the beginning, middle, or end of a program. The applicability of the concepts of death and dying to all areas of nursing might be lost if one separate course were offered. Moreover, if the course were taught under the auspices of a department other than nursing, the essential content related to nursing care might be neglected.

MULTIDISCIPLINARY EDUCATION

In recent years a trend toward multidisciplinary or interdisciplinary education has emerged. Its value lies in sharing significant information of mutual concern across professional boundaries and thereby increasing mutual respect. In order for this to happen there must be a change of attitudes, values, and behaviors for faculty accustomed to working solely within their specialty field. Toward this goal, the University of California at San Francisco has initiated an innovative course for medical students entitled Introduction to Nursing. Death and dying is also in need of multidisciplinary education. Many institutions already teach death-related issues in a multidisciplinary framework. As more multidisciplinary courses are offered, the "team" approach may become something more than a token acknowledgment of the value of each discipline's information and contribution.

In addition to death and dying, other ideas in this book are appropriate to interdisciplinary education. Client's rights are not solely the purview of nurses, but the responsibility of all health care personnel. The well model also needs to be understood and utilized by all health care personnel.

CRISIS INTERVENTION

Throughout this book the elements of crisis and the many situations in which it can occur, not the least of which is dying—the final crisis—have been identified. The fundamental nature of the hospital setting produces many such potential and actual crisis situations, but these are not always noticed because the nurse—the person most likely to be available when a crisis occurs—lacks information and skills in crisis intervention. Crisis theory is usually not taught to nursing students but is seen as applicable to graduate-level education, such as the preparation of psychiatric nurse practitioners. Surely, if volunteers on hotlines can learn crisis intervention, nurses can learn it also. All nurses should be taught the basics of crisis theory and intervention relatively early in their basic program, and in fact, students should be encouraged to work in a crisis-intervention center or on a hotline.

DETERMINANTS OF THE PROGRAM

1 *Previous experience of the participant*   Most people have experienced their first death before their teens. This first death and its resolution have a critical effect on subsequent encounters with the dying process, both professional and personal. With more life experiences and opportunity for grief, the older student's class participation can provoke fruitful discussion. This is not to say that the older student may handle the situation better; he or she may have learned only how to avoid uncomfortable situations and hide feelings.

2 *Expressed needs of the participants*   Any program on death and dying needs to be flexible enough to incorporate the expressed needs of the learners. These can be determined by a questionnaire given out before the first class meeting. This approach provides students with a preliminary opportunity for introspection and stimulates initial class discussion. The teacher, too, has time to make the necessary adjustments in course plans. Another alternative would be to take time in the first class meeting to complete the questionnaire and discuss its implications.

3 *Number of hours allotted to course*   Understanding the concepts of death and dying requires more than reading and discussing Kübler-Ross's stages of dying. Therefore, in-service educational seminars of just 1 or 2 days cannot hope to provide a thorough understanding of the dying client, much less explore the many thorny side issues, such as frank discussion of diagnosis with a client. A course on death and dying requires a full semester for a general grasp of the issues. Concepts and issues of death and dying need periodic review, just as cardiopulmonary resuscitation review is repeated in schools of nursing and in-service educational seminars.

4 *Availability of resources*   To supplement basic lectures and class discussions there must be adequate outside resources, such as a library with books about death and dying. Guest lecturers from many fields add breadth and a change of pace from the usual lecturer. A check of local resources, including schools offering clinical pastoral education and health care personnel working in various capacities such as crisis intervention, might provide valuable people.

Many kinds of excellent audiovisual materials, such as films, film loops, filmstrips, cassettes, audiotapes, videotapes, slides, records, and games, are available, many with teachers' guides. Appendix B provides a partial listing of the distributors. These resources are limited only by the imagination of the instructor. A good way to begin a class and establish a mood is by using art or literature, for example, slides of works of art depicting a death-related concept or an appropriate recitation from literature. Both contemporary and older music can set a mood and illustrate the preoccupation with death in our lives. Slides of death as a natural process might include autumnal or winter scenes or dead animals. Slides of violent, accidental or volitional, single or mass deaths also stimulate thought and conversation. Sometimes an allegory may be helpful.

5 *Faculty preparation*   Death and dying has only in recent years been included in the nursing curriculum, and still remains a rarity in the medical school curriculum. Much of the success of a course depends upon the knowledge, creativity, and personal qualities of the instructor. A broad understanding of issues and concepts and clinical experience in the care of the dying is essential. The instructor does not have to be a psychiatric nursing specialist but should have knowledge of counseling and crisis-intervention techniques.

Teachers have as difficult a time coping with the dying as do students. Unless faculty in-service education addresses the needs of the dying client, nursing personnel will continue to perpetuate the same mistakes. Faculty as well as practitioners also react to death personally before they react professionally with job titles and responsibilities. (Figure 8-1). The problem of educating the faculty on death is fourfold: One, the taboo of death still exists. Two, support systems must be established within the structure of the school. Three, outside support and counseling is sometimes needed during particularly stressful times. Four, faculty must provide counseling of individual students as needed.

The taboo of death presumably has been broken with the recent wide dissemination of information about the subject, but in many ways it, as well as sex, has retained its unspeakable nature. Until recently nurses were taught only postmortem care. Many schools of nursing still have no death education course.

Kron mentions a nurse instructor who resigned her position because the faculty did not approve of her teaching death and dying to freshman students.

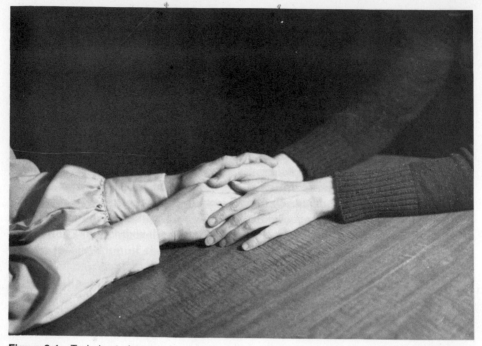

Figure 8-1 To help students understand how to care for dying clients, the teacher not only gives information but also shares in self-growth through mutual vulnerability.

Another example combines both the death and the sex taboo. A junior student, a woman in her forties, married, with three children, chose, as part of a project in operating room nursing, to invite a controversial abortion advocate to lecture to her class. Permission to attend was granted to all but the freshmen, ostensibly because abortion was not relevant to their program. The freshman year does not include maternal and child health or operating room nursing, two areas in which abortion is relevant. This story illustrates the effect deep-seated attitudes about death and sex have on how and what is taught to whom. This is not an example of bureaucratic decision making.

Once the faculty are able to handle the fact that they, too, have fears and negative attitudes about dying, they must recognize the need for continuous mutual support. Just as staff nurses in the acutely and chronically dying settings, mentioned in Chapters 6 and 7, need built-in supports, so do the faculty. Administrative support is essential. Periodic breaks from classroom and clinical responsibilities are necessary to regain perspective and to prevent overload. In addition, regular group meetings with an outside person such as a psychologist, social worker, psychiatrist, or clergy, as mentioned in Chapters 6 and 7, are also helpful for faculty.

Outside support and counseling of individuals are sometimes necessary too. The death educator is responsible for course content; process; and the unforeseen, unavailable, unfortunate, and unpleasant repercussions. Leviton, for instance, points out that suicide is always a possibility in especially prone individuals when a topic is raised about which they have suppressed terror.

When a suicide occurs, the instructor must then find a way to work through the subsequent guilt feelings and the fear of recriminations from news media and citizens' groups.

Faculty must anticipate students' difficulties and provide appropriate individual counseling when necessary. In "studying" death students may go through the same emotions as the dying person. The intense emotional reactions may be more than a student can handle, especially if he or she is depressed, has family problems, or has a dying family member. The death educator must be sophisticated in both counseling and crisis intervention and be available at regularly scheduled office hours. Leviton cites three major reasons for students seeking counseling during a death education course: (1) concern over impending or past death of a loved one, (2) suicidal thinking, and (3) thanatophobia, or preoccupation with fears of personal death.

6 *Clinical facilities and experience*   Classroom discussion, readings, and other modalities are essential to clarify issues and values relating to death and dying. Both the cognitive and the affective levels can be addressed in this "safe" environment. Epstein suggests that simulation training in the classroom may help to avoid mistakes, trauma, guilt, and self-doubt when the nurse is in an actual clinical situation. It may even be possible intellectually to develop an ideal approach to death and dying in the classroom. Without clinical experience, though, death and dying is all talk. It is in the clinical setting that the conflicts inherent in the care of the dying can erupt into very painful experiences or can be a rewarding challenge.

Early in their education student nurses are introduced to death in the anatomical dissecting class. it is here that they begin to learn to be objective. Gradually in the clinical setting they care for clients needing increasingly complex knowledge and skills. If a student is assigned to a dying client, Quint states, it is primarily for other reasons, such as an interesting diagnosis or a new procedure. Instructors may also not even identify a dying client as such, especially in the preterminal phases of dying.

The client who is not identified as dying and really is poses a threat for the unprepared student. The client may suddenly "go bad," want to talk about dying, or display baffling behavior. If the nurse realizes that the client is (1) dying or (2) feeling that his or her life is threatened, the client's behavior, in reacting to loss and anticipatory grief, is much more understandable. Therefore, clients in different phases of dying provide valuable learning experiences.

Because of the nature of each program and the kinds of clients available, there are certain constraints on any course. A variety of experiences can be obtained by frequent rotation to different floors in a hospital, but as much as this provides opportunities to care for a variety of clients under different situations, the length of time spent with any one client may be severely limited. Relationships and rapport with clients take time to develop. The number of hours per day and number of days per week can also hinder prolonged client contact. In addition, the kind of hospital available affects the student's clinical experience. The chronic disease hospital provides kinds of opportunities different from those provided by the emergency ward or obstetrical unit of a general hospital. The student needs to care for a variety of clients in different phases of dying, both acute and chronic, over long periods of time.

In a school using the adult education model, students may choose their own clients. There are real advantages to this student choice of assignment. Students can pace themselves, which is especially necessary in caring for dying clients. Of course, this arrangement does not eliminate all possibilities of awkward or traumatic encounters, but it may help reduce some of the anxiety students feel in caring for the dying client.

TOPICS FOR COURSE

This section presents broad topics for discussion relevant to nurses at various levels. Except for the first topic, they are not presented in any hierarchical or chronological order. The objectives of the program, level and interest of the learner, and time and resources available will determine the applicability, depth, and priority of topics. From a pedagogical standpoint it is essential that learning behaviors be explicitly stated. The style in which the class is conducted should also be stated. This may vary depending upon the topic. An atmosphere of openness, discussion, and acceptance of feelings is essential throughout the course.

The previous chapters in this book can be well integrated into the entire course. Readings listed at the end of each chapter also provide pertinent information. Although not exhaustive, these suggestions are a good beginning. (It is impossible, due to the volume of information on death and dying currently in print, to be complete.) In addition, the questions for reflection at the end of each chapter are good exercises and discussion topics.

I   Introduction and expression of feelings
   A   Rationale
       Introductory remarks should fulfill three objectives. First, to get the learners to begin thinking about death and dying, a discussion of cultural and societal factors affecting the death taboo is appropriate. How society views death and dying provides necessary background for why death education is needed. Second, to establish an atmosphere conducive to free expression of feelings, it is necessary to first recognize the role personal feelings play in nursing. Values and attitudes affect nursing care. (The students should express their own specific needs and goals for the course.) Three, to identify the direction of the course and establish responsibility of students in terms of assignments and class participation, course requirements should be specified.
   B   Methods
       1   Discuss societal and cultural views of death: other cultures, old and new; use of euphemisms; and death taboo.
       2   Show films.
           a   Personal-account films such as *How Could I Not Be Among You?* (distributed by the Eccentric Circle Cinema Workshop)
           b   Cultural views of death such as *Day of the Dead* (distributed by the Charles Eames Office)
       3   Distribute pre- and postcourse questionnaires like Shneidman's, Seeland's, Epstein's, or Nursing 75's. These questionnaires can

be used to relate to a specific issue, such as euthanasia, or to identify personal attitudes and values. Changes in attitudes and values as a result of maturation and course content can be identified.

4   Have students draw a picture of death. Each student draws a picture of death and describes it for the class. This can be done in large and small groups and is effective in illustrating that there are many viewpoints about death.

5   Students can write own obituary, eulogy, death certificate, and tombstone inscription.

6   Have students complete death-word puzzle. This technique familiarizes students with noneuphemistic language.

7   Relate death fantasy. Described by Kopel, this exercise asks participants to imagine themselves as isolated natural disaster victims with a very short time to live. The task in small groups is to assist each other to die with dignity. Sharing imminent death with a stranger is likened to the dying client's sharing thoughts with a nurse.

8   Use finger paint. This is a very effective nonverbal way for both adults and children to describe personal feelings about death, especially when words cannot convey the depth of feeling.

9   Assign readings.
    a   Chapter 1 of this book
    b   Any personal-account narrative, such as Alsop's *Stay of Execution*
    c   Fulton and Langton's "Attitudes toward Death: An Emerging Mental Health Problem"

C   Questions for classroom discussion
    (Refer to Chapter 1's Questions for Reflection and Discussion)
    1   Why did you become a nurse? This may sound trite but it is very relevant to nurses' views of themselves. Dying clients can sometimes strip nurses of their ideal view of themselves.
    2   If you were told you had a terminal illness and had a limited time to live, how would you want to spend your time until you died?
    3   How do you want other people to act when you die?
    4   From what culture do you come? How are your beliefs about dying affected by your cultural background?

II   Definitions of death
   A   Rationale
       Over the years the criteria for diagnosis of death have changed. Legally, only the physician can declare a person dead, but the word *dead* is much more than a pronouncement by the physician. The way it is understood by the public and the health professions has personal and societal ramifications. For nurses, a course on death and dying must teach not just actual care of the dying but also the various kinds of deaths and their influences on how care is given.
   B   Method
       1   Discuss kinds of death.
           a   *Social*   The old, ugly, deformed, retarded, unconscious, der-

elict, and institutionalized are sometimes thought of as socially dead.

    b *Cultural* Whole societies, for example, ancient Rome, have died.

    c *Biological* Cells, organs, systems, and whole bodies die. Discuss the impact of biological death on organ donation.

    d *Physiological* Formerly it was cardiac arrest, but now the cessation of cortical activity (based on the Harvard definition) is the usual definition of physiological death.

    e *Legal* This is based on the medical, or physiological, definition of death. A physician is the only person who can determine this. Discuss court cases involving termination of life.

    f *Psychological* Motives underlying dying have an effect on how a person dies. Discuss homicide, suicide, subintentioned death, and many others. Discuss psychological autopsy.

    g *Appropriate* Weisman discusses the concept of appropriate death in relation to individual wishes and needs. An appropriate death may be different for each person.

  2 Invite guest lecturers, such as a lawyer and a sociologist.

  3 Discuss current newspaper topics relating to kinds of death.

  4 Assign readings.

    a *Social* Sudnow, Mendelson, and Glaser and Strauss cited earlier; Fox's *Experiment Perilous*

    b *Cultural* Bronowski cited earlier

    c *Biological* Williams cited earlier

    d *Physiological* White, "The Scientific Limitations of Brain Death"; "Diagnosis of Death"; and Veatch, "The Whole-Brain Oriented Concept of Death: An Outmoded Philosophical Formulation"

    e *Legal* Hendin, Mannes, and Williams cited earlier

    f *Psychological* Shneidman's *Deaths of Man* and "Orientations toward Death: A Vital Aspect of the Study of Lives" Weisman and Kastenbaum's *The Psychological Autopsy: A Study of the Terminal Phase of Life*, and Weisman's *The Realization of Death*

    g *Appropriate* Weisman cited earlier

 C Questions for classroom discussion

  1 Does society have a responsibility to the socially dead? If so, what is it?

  2 What is the role of the nurse in postdeath care of the client and family?

  3 What would be an appropriate death for you?

  4 What is the difference between subintentioned death and suicide?

  5 What does the psychological autopsy seek to prove?

III Religious aspects of death

 A Rationale

Not every person expresses religious needs and feelings during the dying process, but the nurse needs to assist clients who do wish to have religious support. The value of clergy for many people cannot be underestimated. Some clergy provide primarily the ritual associated with dying, while others also act as pastoral counselors.

  B Method

    1 Discuss theological concepts relating to death and dying and the way individual philosophies and religious beliefs affect the dying process.

    2 Use clergy, from Protestant, Catholic, and Jewish faiths for example, as guest lecturers.

    3 Show films.

      a *The Day Grandpa Died* (distributed by the Bailey Film Association) illustrates Jewish tradition

      b *Walk up the Hill* (distributed by Church Films) depicts the Christian viewpoint

    4 Assign readings: Grollman cited earlier.

  C Questions for classroom discussion

    1 Do you believe it is appropriate for the nurse to discuss religious beliefs with a dying person?

    2 How do you make a conversation meaningful if your religious beliefs differ from those of the client?

    3 How do you plan for and work with a chaplain in providing for spiritual care of the dying client?

IV Death and the funeral: Rites and rituals

  A Rationale

They may begin with the family gathering around the dying person's bed, and custom determines when and how they end, but rituals surrounding death exist to some degree in all cultures. The funeral is the major rite of passage. In the United States recently, less stress has been placed on the ritualistic part of dying, but the nurse should understand the purpose and value of the rituals to the dying person and family. For some dying clients and their families, part of the resolution of anticipatory grief occurs as they plan the funeral. The two major purposes of the funeral are (1) to publicly acknowledge the death and (2) to provide for appropriate expressions of grief by mourners.

  B Method

    1 Discuss topics such as how to assist the family during acute grief, funerals, memorial services, burial societies, and wills.

    2 Invite such guest speakers as a funeral director.

    3 Show film *Dead Man* (distributed by Foundation of Thanatology), which depicts the stark reality of death.

    4 Assign further learning experiences.

      a Viewing an autopsy

      b Submitting a report (oral or written, single or group) of interviews of people who do postdeath work, such as morticians, funeral directors, coroners, morgue workers, and students in embalming school. Tour their places of work. In the report the following questions should be answered:

        (1) Why have they chosen this kind of work?

        (2) How are they prepared for their work?

(3)   What kinds of tasks does their work entail?
(4)   What kinds of feelings do they have about their work, especially about the difficult aspects?
5   Assign readings.
   a   Grollman and Mitford previously cited
   b   Mandelbaum's "Social Uses of Funeral Rites"
C   Questions for classroom discussion
   1   Are wills necessary?
   2   What purpose does preplanning a funeral serve?
   3   Is embalming required by law?
   4   What is the difference between a coroner and a medical examiner? What are their duties?
   5   How should a cemetery be chosen?
   6   What are the relative costs of funerals and memorials?
   7   What are the advantages and disadvantages of cremation?
   8   What are memorial societies and how do they function?
V   Aging
   A   Rationale
   A large portion of our population is over 65 years of age; all must face death. How one faces death depends in part on how one has lived. The current negative stereotype of the older person in America has a deleterious effect on how the older person lives and dies. Nurses must understand the needs of the elderly and help change the negative stereotype.
   B   Method
      1   Invite guest speakers from volunteer senior citizens' groups such as Gray Panthers to talk about the work they do.
      2   Show film such as *Joy of Love* (distributed by the University of Michigan AV Center), which depicts the life and memories of an elderly widower.
      3   Assign further learning experiences.
         a   Submit report (oral or written, single or group) on one of the following topics:
            (1)   Visit places frequented by older persons: senior citizens' meetings, nursing homes, acute and chronic care hospitals, hot lunch programs and housing projects (especially senior citizen housing projects). Visit a homebound elderly person. Find out (1) things elderly persons enjoy in life, (2) problems, and (3) fears now and for the future.
            (2)   Ask 10 people of various backgrounds over 65 years of age (1) the last time they received health care, (2) where they received it, (3) where, to whom, and how often do they receive primary health care, and (4) how much of this health care Medicare and Medicaid pay for?
            (3)   Visit local department of elderly affairs. Find out ways the community helps older people financially (for instance, some localities have discounts for public transportation and stores) and socially.
            (4)   Find out procedure for applying for food stamps. How

long does it take? Do any of the people you interviewed in items 1 and 2 receive food stamps? What percentage of people receiving food stamps are over 65 years of age?

    b Assign readings: Chapter 7, section on aging; Butler and Busser cited earlier

C Questions for classroom discussion
(Refer to Chapter 7's Questions for Reflection and Discussion, which include many aspects of aging in America.)

    1 Do you as an individual have a responsibility to the older person?

    2 Does society as a whole have a responsibility to the older person?

    3 What are some of the losses an older person experiences?

    4 What are some of the possible reasons for fear of death in youth, adolescence, middle age, and old age?

    5 How can an older person remain active and useful? In the face of chronic illness too?

    6 What factors have contributed to the negative stereotype of old age?

    7 How can this negative stereotype be overcome by you individually and by society at large?

    8 Are there any alternatives to nursing home care for older persons unable to care for themselves?

VI Loss, grief, mourning, bereavement

  A Rationale
Loss and grief are universal phenomena. Nurses care for many clients with various kinds of losses in different phases of resolution. Therefore, they should understand the dynamics of grief, the time it takes to resolve it, and the appropriate nursing intervention.

  B Method

    1 Discuss Engle's, Kübler-Ross's, and Lindemann's grief concepts. Relate loss also to body-image change, chronic illness, and crisis.

    2 Use stage chart to compare theorists.

    3 Follow Epstein's specific exercises to help identify where in the grieving process the client, family, and nurse are.

    4 Invite guest speakers from volunteer programs such as:

      a Widow-to-Widow Program—bereavement

      b Make Today Count—anticipatory grief

      c Ostomy clubs—body-image change; anticipatory grief

      d Suicide prevention centers—profound loss

    5 Show film such as *Until I Die* (distributed by American Journal of Nursing Film Library), describing Kübler-Ross's five stages. Other films and audiocassettes are available in which she describes her theory.

    6 Invite a professional guest speaker, such as a psychiatrist, psychiatric nurse, or social worker, doing individual or group therapy with chronically dying persons and bereaved families.

    7 Assign further learning experiences.

      a Submit report (oral or written, single or group) on the following research: Attend a meeting of any of the volunteer organizations in item 4. Interview the participants. Find out (a) why they are there and (b) what ways the organization helps them cope with loss or impending loss.

 b Work in a crisis-intervention center to learn the basic techniques.

 8 Role play situations to help the student develop appropriate responses to clients and their families.

 9 Assign readings

 a Chapters 5, 6, and 7 include information about grief, body image, loss, and crisis

 b References cited throughout this book refer to these concepts; some examples: Peretz, Norris, Crate, Aguilera, Engle, Gullo, Kübler-Ross, and Lindemann

C Questions for classroom discussion

 (Refer to Chapters 2 and 5's Questions for Reflection and Discussion)

 1 Does the nurse have any role to play in mourning and grief?

 2 At what age are people most afraid of death?

 3 What kinds of losses does the person who is dying experience?

 4 How does the nurse identify these losses?

 5 How does hospitalization provide for or impinge on the grieving process of the client and family?

VII Nurse's role

A Rationale

 With all the advancements in medicine, clients still die. As caregivers, nurses play a crucial role in the process. Even for nurses who choose to work in a unit with a low death rate, clients still die. The quality of care—not just the technical care, but also the human component of compassion—can significantly alter the degree of comfort or discomfort experienced by the client.

B Method

 1 Discuss the care versus cure conflict, telling truthful diagnosis, nurse's relationship with other health care personnel including doctor, communication techniques (especially how to listen), problems of nurses in acute and chronic settings, and positive approaches to overcoming conflicts.

 2 Invite nurse clinical specialists in thanatology to give guest lectures.

 3 Show film on nursing care of the dying. (Many are available.)

 4 Role play nurse-client interactions on a variety of dying-related subjects. Refer to Barton and Crowder. Since the instructor is asking students to risk exposure of their feelings, the instructor might also take a role-playing part to show that he or she is willing also to be exposed.

 5 Present psychodrama. Many kinds of situations can be explored using psychodrama, but the instructor needs special preparation. Refer to Weiner.

 6 Use self- or programmed instructional units. Refer to Koenig.

 7 Assign further learning experiences.

 a Submit report (oral or written, single or group): Interview five physicians of varying backgrounds. Find out (1) what does each see as the most difficult problem for the physician in handling death? (2) What death does each remember most vividly? Why? (3) What is the philosophy of each regarding revealing a fatal diagnosis? (4) What does each think is the nurse's most difficult problem in the care of dying clients? During your conversations were there any communication difficulties? If so, what happened and what were your reactions? How did you handle the situation?

b Care for a chronically dying client over a long period of time. Spend time with the person for discussion about what is important to him or her. Find out the person's (1) present and future concerns, (2) awareness context, (3) view of relationships with family, and (4) views of the institution and staff providing care. Identify your feelings about him or her and the relationship you established. Make notes of your conversation, or use process recording to describe changes in behavior, feelings, and conversation taking place over time. Did conversation become easier or more difficult as time progressed? What conversations and in what situations were you most comfortable? How did you handle them? What conversations and situations were easiest? Why?

c Care for an acutely dying client. Answer the same questions as asked in 7b. About what aspects of this client and his or her care were you unable to find information? Did the need for physical care ever interfere with conversation or psychological care of the client? Were there any uncomfortable times for you? Why and what happened?

d Write paper (single page) on "Philosophy of Living and Dying." Explain your philosophy of nursing as a service to people. Consider clients' human right to choose the way they live and die and society's mandate to set and enforce rules and regulations for the common good. How do you plan now and in the future to implement this philosophy? What barriers might prevent you from accomplishing or make it more difficult for you to accomplish your goal? What steps must you take? What risks must be faced? How does all this relate to the dying client?

8 Assign readings.
   a Chapters 6 and 7, especially as related to nurse's conflicts
   b Glaser and Strauss cited earlier
   c Quint cited earlier

C Questions for classroom discussion
   (Refer to Chapters 6 and 7's Questions for Reflection and Discussion.)
   1 How do you feel when your client dies? Relate a specific instance in both the acute and the chronic setting.
   2 How is terminal care of the cancer client different from and similar to care of the client with an acute myocardial infarction? How can you meet these needs?
   3 How can the nursing team provide the environment for death that a client desires?

4 At what point does cure care end and comfort care begin? Who makes that decision?

5 What is your responsibility in discussing death with a client?

6 How do you cope with your personal feelings about the death of a particular client? Give an example.

7 How can dealing with death be a total nursing involvement?

8 How do you maintain a person's hope and at the same time remain honest about dying?

9 What are the responsibilities of the nurse after a death has occurred?

10 Does the nurse have a responsibility to the bereaved family after the death has occurred? If so, how long does this responsibility extend?

11 In what ways is death a difficult occupational problem for physicians?

VIII Family's role

   A Rationale

The death of a client has repercussions for the whole family structure. Individually and collectively the family grieves in anticipation of death. Often this grief is not synchronized with that of the client. The degree of dissonance sometimes makes communication even more difficult. Just as the nurse has a role in client care, so also does the nurse have a role in assisting the family.

   B Method

     1 Discuss family interaction and developmental aspects of dying: dying for the child, adolescent, and adult; how to talk to children about dying.

     2 Invite a guest speaker.

       a Counselor of individual family members or groups

       b Family member of a dying client

       c Member of Cancer Care, Inc., in New York. This organization stresses maintaining family integrity during catastrophic illness.

     3 Show film on dynamics of family interaction and positive value of maintaining optimal communication.

     4 Role play nurse and family-member interactions. This approach can produce new avenues to solving communications problems in particular.

     5 Assign further learning experiences.

       a Submit report (oral or written, single or group) on the following topic: Interview family members of a dying client. Find out (1) their fears, (2) how they cope, and (3) how they support the client

       b Ask three children, one each at ages 3 to 4, 5 to 7, and 8 to 10, what death means to them. Compare your results with Nagy's developmental stages.

     6 Assign readings.

       a Chapters 2, 4, 6, and 7 as they relate to family members

       b Grollman and Schoenberg et al. cited earlier

       c Nagy and Gullo

C   Questions for classroom discussion
   1   Have you observed others talking to children about death? What approach works best?
   2   How would you develop a plan of emotional care for the dying child? How would this plan differ for an adult?
   3   What are your responsibilities to the children of a dying parent?
   4   When should a child be told a parent is dying?
   5   How can the nursing team provide the environment for death that family and friends desire?
   6   What is your responsibility in discussing death with the dying client's family and friends?
   7   How can the hospital provide more privacy for family interaction during visiting hours?
   8   Does the hospital have a responsibility for providing privacy for fulfilling of sexual needs between dying client and significant other?

IX   Euthanasia
  A   Rationale
    Technology has provided the health professions with the expertise to prolong a persons' life, sometimes indefinitely. Since the nurse does not function in a vacuum but practices within an ethical and moral framework, the quality of the client's thus prolonged life must be considered. The decisions made are based on why, for what purpose, and for what good care is being given. Finally, who should make the life-prolonging or death-delaying decisions? The client? The physician? All these issues need to be considered by nurses caring for the dying. The solutions are not easy to determine.
  B   Method
   1   Invite a speaker from the Euthanasia Educational Council to discuss the Living Will.
   2   Show film (or short excerpts) relating to euthanasia.
   3   Debate pros and cons of euthanasia, suicide, and abortion. Discuss court cases involving termination of life.
   4   Assign further learning experiences.
     a   Submit report (oral or written, single or group) on one of the following topics:
       (1)   Observe in a hemodialysis center. Discuss with clients the quality of their lives. Describe their activities of daily living. What are your feelings?
       (2)   Observe at a suicide prevention center. Describe the kinds of clients seen at this center. What are your feelings?
     b   Assign readings: Williams and Mannes cited earlier
  C   Questions for classroom discussion
   1   What is dignity in dying?
   2   How does the nurse provide the client with dignity in dying?
   3   What are some of the reasons a terminally ill client might desire to die or might wish to live longer?

4 How could you find out what aspects of death are most distasteful to your client? How could you then assist?

5 Was there a time in your life when you wanted to die? When? What were the circumstances?

6 If you had a choice, what kind of death would you prefer?

7 What is "appropriate" death?

8 How do the media report examples of dying or euthanasia?

9 What are negative and positive euthanasia?

X Clients' rights

  A Rationale

Dying clients have a human right to compassionate care and an appropriate death. The nurse must carefully respect these rights. Because clients may not be physically or emotionally strong enough or may not know their rights, the nurse often must be their advocate.

  B Method

    1 Invite guest speaker, for instance, lawyer knowledgeable about clients' and institutions' rights. The hospital and the client are adversaries in some situations.

    2 Show film, for example, *The Lyn Helton Story* (distributed by Oregon Division of Continuing Education Film Library), about clients' right to refuse care.

    3 Role play many "rights" situations.

      a A disgruntled client insists on having the construction noise outside his room stopped, but the hospital cannot stop it.

      b A client wants to sign out of the hospital against medical advice.

      c A client refuses medication.

    4 Assign readings.

      a Several medical-legal periodicals

      b Creighton, who has much legal information useful for the nurse

      c Chapters 3 and 5 of this book as related to rights

  C Questions for classroom discussion

(Refer to Chapter 2's Questions for Reflection and Discussion on clients' rights.)

    1 Does your hospital have a client representative? What does this person do? Is this a voluntary or paid position? If paid, who provides this person's salary?

    2 How are the rights of terminal and nonterminal clients different and the same?

    3 In your state, what is the legal status of clients' right to see their charts?

    4 How does the hospital system deny clients their rights?

    5 How do you give clients more choice in their living and dying?

    6 Ask a client what he or she understands about signing his consent form.

    7 When is the best time for a client to sign a consent form for a major procedure? Just before the procedure, or days before?

    8 Make a list of the ways and number of times clients' privacy is

invaded and interrupted. How can you protect their privacy in the future?

XI   Alternatives to acute hospital care

   A   Rationale

The acute hospital is recovery-or-cure-oriented and operates on the sick model. For the dying client it may be an inappropriate place for various reasons. When at home, many chronically dying clients spend most of their time living to their maximum ability, that is, functioning on the well model. The acute care hospital is appropriate for treatment of exacerbations and for prophylactic chemotherapy. Even chemotherapy is often given on an outpatient basis. In fact, there are alternatives to the acute care hospital, and more are needed.

   B   Method

      1   Discuss advantages and disadvantages of the acute hospital care.

      2   Show film *Dignity of Death* (distributed by ABC News), about St. Christopher's Hospice in London.

      3   Show slides of the hospice in New Haven, Connecticut.

      4   Invite guest speaker discussing practical aspects of home care and family's role.

         a   Member of Cancer Care, Inc.

         b   Representative of Visiting Nurse Service

      5   Assign further learning experiences.

         a   Submit report (oral or written, single) on the following topic: Visit the home of a dying client with a visiting nurse. Find out (1) life-style, (2) ways client and family cope, (3) problems, and (4) support systems.

         b   Assign readings: Chapter 7, section on home versus institutional care; readings at end of Chapter 7

   C   Questions for classroom discussion

      1   Why is the acute care hospital often an inappropriate place for care of the chronically dying client?

      2   What are the advantages of places like St. Christopher's Hospice?

      3   Would a client ever choose an acute hospital as opposed to home care? Explain possible reasons.

      4   For the client who chooses to die at home, what preparation is needed by the family?

      5   While the client is being cared for at home, how can the nurse and health team support both client and family emotionally?

XII Pain control

   A   Rationale

Aside from dependency and loss of loved ones, the most fearful part of dying, for many clients, is pain. The nurse plays a pivotal role in pain relief.

   B   Method

      1   Discuss the following topics related to pain.

         a   Pathophysiology and affective and cultural responses to pain

         b   Techniques: acupuncture, biofeedback, hypnosis, surgical procedures, and others

      c Drugs: narcotic and non-narcotic analgesics, alcohol, heroin, and mood-altering drugs

      d Recording of a pain history

      e Evaluation of a client's pain response

  2 Show film *Pain! Where Does It Hurt?* (distributed by NCB Educational Enterprises), describing newer experimental pain-relief methods.

  3 Role play a situation in which a client in pain is given medication that is ineffective.

  4 Invite guest speakers to demonstrate acupuncture, biofeedback, hypnosis, etc.

  5 Assign further learning experiences.

      a Submit report (oral or written, single or group) on one of the following topics:

          (1) Visit acupuncture, hypnosis, or pain clinic and find out (a) theory behind the technique, (b) kinds of pain treated, and (c) effectiveness of the technique.

          (2) Take a pain history (use pain section of the strength-oriented nursing record, referred to in Chapter 4) on yourself, on a classmate, then on a client. Compare method of coping, cultural background, and kinds of pain.

      b Select a pain-relief modality and give a short presentation to the class.

      c Assign readings Copp, Gonda, Kübler-Ross, McLachlin, Murray, Weisenberg, McCaffrey, and Davis et al. cited earlier.

C Questions for classroom discussion

  1 Have you ever experienced pain? Describe the circumstances.

  2 What are some cultural stereotypes in regard to pain response?

  3 In what ways does the hospital experience prevent clients from using their own coping responses?

  4 How can the nurse help to overcome the problem in question 3?

  5 Is there any kind of client pain response to which you react negatively, such as moaning?

  6 In what ways is pain legitimized?

  7 In what situations, if any, do you withhold pain medication from a client?

  8 How do you feel about giving pain medication to a client whom you either think or know is addicted?

  9 Is there ever any reason to give a placebo? Are you violating any of the client's rights? What is the result if the client finds out you have given a placebo? What would your reaction be if you found out you had been given a placebo?

SUMMARY

Curriculum guidelines are a skeleton from which a course on death and dying, with integrated well model concepts, can be taught. Death-related concepts can be taught in a separate course or be integrated throughout the program. Integrated concepts allow students to mature gradually in knowledge and feeling and see the usefulness of the issues of death and dying throughout their professional and personal lives. Because the quality of instruction and guidance may vary with teachers, concepts of death and dying may not be uniformly presented. A separate course given by a person with a thorough knowledge of thanatology would provide the depth and consistency needed, but placement of that one course in the curriculum is problematic.

Multidisciplinary education is valuable in teaching death-related issues, crisis, the Well Model, and many other areas because all participants in multidisciplinary education share common problems and insights. It also increases mutual respect among disciplines. Modifications of curriculum guidelines in terms of the expressed needs of the students, number of hours allotted to the course, resources available, faculty preparation, and clinical experience and facilities are of course necessary.

The course materials presented were rationale, teaching methods, and media suggestions as well as readings and discussion questions for each topic. Values and attitudes also integrated throughout the topics include introduction and expression of feelings, definitions of death, religious aspects, funeral rites and rituals, aging, loss, grief, mourning and bereavement, nurse's role, family's role, euthanasia, client's rights, alternatives to acute hospital care, and pain control.

BIBLIOGRAPHY

Alsop, S.: *Stay of Execution*, Philadelphia, J. B. Lippincott Co., 1973.

Arnold, J., et al.: "Public Attitudes and the Diagnosis of Death," *Journal of American Medical Association*, **206**(9):1949–1954, November 25, 1968.

Barton, D., and Crowder, M.: "The Use of Role Playing Techniques as an Instructional Aid in Teaching about Dying, Death and Bereavement," *Omega*, **6**(3):243–250, 1975.

Colton, A., et al.: "A Faculty Workshop on Death Attitudes and Life Affirmation," *Omega*, **4**(1):51–56, 1973.

Creighton, H.: *Law Every Nurse Should Know*, Philadelphia, W. B. Saunders Co., 1970.

"Diagnosis of Death," *Ames Diagnostica*, **22**:6–11, February 1972.

Duke, P.: "Media on Death and Dying," *Omega*, **6**(3):275–287, 1975.

Earle, A., et al. (ed.): *The Nurse as Caregiver for the Terminal Patient and His Family*, New York, Columbia University Press, 1976.

Epstein, C.: *Nursing the Dying Patient, Learning Processes for Interaction*, Reston, Va., Reston Publishing Co., 1975.

Folck, M., and Nie, P.: "Nursing Students Learn to Face Death," *Nursing Outlook*, **7**(9):510–513, September 1959.

Fox, R.: *Experiment Perilous*, Glencoe, Ill., Free Press of Glencoe, 1959.

Fulton, R., and Langton, P.: "Attitudes toward Death: An Emerging Mental Health Problem," *Nursing Forum*, **3**(1):105–112.

Gullo, S.: "Games Children Play when They are Dying," *Medical Dimensions*, 23–28, October 1973.

Harding, E., et al.: "A Nursing Course for Medical Students," *Nursing Outlook*, **23**(4):240–242, April 1975.

Kelly, O.: "Make Today Count," in Feifel, H. (ed.), *New Meanings of Death*, New York, McGraw-Hill Book Co., 1977, pp. 182–193.

Koenig, R.: "Counseling in Catastrophic Illness: A Self-Instructional Unit," *Omega*, **6**(3):227–241, 1975.

Kopel, K., et al.: "A Human Relations Laboratory Approach to Death and Dying," *Omega*, **6**(3):219–221, 1975.

Kron, J.: "Learning to Live with Death," *Omega*, **5**(1):5–24, 1974.

Leviton, D.: "Education for Death, or Death Becomes Less a Stranger," *Omega*, **6**(3):183–191, 1975.

Liston, E.: "Education on Death and Dying: A Neglected Area in the Medical Curriculum," *Omega*, **6**(3):193–198, 1975.

Mandelbaum, D.: "Social Uses of Funeral Rites," in Feifel, H. (ed.), *The Meaning of Death*, New York, McGraw-Hill Book Co., 1959.

Mills, G., et al.: *Discussing Death, a Guide to Death Education*, Homewood, Ill., ETC Publications, 1976.

Nagy, M.: "The Child's View of Death," in Feifel, H. (ed.), *The Meaning of Death*, New York, McGraw-Hill Book Co., 1959.

Popoff, D.: "What Are Your Feelings about Death and Dying?" *Nursing 74:* Pt. I, **5**(8):15–24, August 1975; Pt. II, **5**(9):55–62, September 1975; Pt. III, **5**(10):39–50, October 1975.

Quint, J.: *The Nurse and the Dying Patient*, New York, Macmillan Co., 1967.

———, and Strauss, A.: "Nursing Students, Assignments and Patients," *Nursing Outlook*, **12**(1):24–27, January 1964.

Sanford, N., and Deloughery, G.: "Teaching Nurses to Care for the Dying Patient," *Journal of Psychiatric Nursing and Mental Health Services*, 24–26, January–February 1973.

Shneidman, E.: *Deaths of Man*, Baltimore, Penguin Books, 1973.

———: "Orientations toward Death: A Vital Aspect of the Study of Lives," in Resnick, H., (ed.), *Suicidal Behavior*, Boston, Little, Brown and Co., 1968.

———: "You and Death Questionnaire," *Psychology Today*, **4**(3):67, 1970.

Seeland, I.: "Attitudes toward Death, Dying, and Bereavement. Surveys of Various Disciplines," *Archives of the Foundation of Thanatology*, **5**(4):405–410, 1975.

Silverman, P.: *"The Widow-to-Widow Program: An Experiment in Preventive Intervention*, in Shneidman, E. (ed.), *Death: Current Perspectives*, Palo Alto, Calif., Mayfield Publishing Co., 1976.

Strauss, A., and Glaser, B.: *Anguish, A Case History of a Dying Trajectory*, Mill Valley, Calif., Sociology Press, 1970.

Veatch, R.: "The Whole-Brain Oriented Concept of Death: An Outmoded Philosophical Formulation," *Journal of Thanatology*, **3**:13–30, 1975.

Weiner, H.: Living Experiences with Death—A Journeyman's View through Psychodrama," *Omega*, **6**(3):251–273, 1975.

Weisman, A.: *The Realization of Death*, New York, Jason Aronson, 1974.

———, and Kastenbaum, R.: *The Psychological Autopsy: A Study of the Terminal Phase of Life*, Community Mental Health Journal Monograph No. 4, New York, Behavioral Publications, 1968.

White, R.: "The Scientific Limitations of Brain Death," *Hospital Progress*, 48–51, March 1972.

Wieczorek, R., Pennington, E., and Fields, S.: "Interdisciplinary Education, A Model for the Resocialization of Faculty," *Nursing Forum*, **15**(3):224–237, 1976.

Wise, D.: "Learning about Dying," *Nursing Outlook*, **22**(1):42–43, January 1974.

Citizens Bill of Hospital Rights: What the Patient and Public Can and Should Expect from Our Hospitals

Author's note: Even though it is now customary to do so, if a hospital adopts a client's Bill of Rights, the American Hospital Association document is used. The Denenberg document presented here was the model for the modified one of the American Hospital Association.

This document is the first one elaborating in detail a client's rights to be published by a government agency. Surely this is a step in the right direction. The crux of the remaining problem is implementation and consumer control.

1 *Quality care* The public has a right to good quality care and high professional standards that are continuously monitored and reviewed. This includes frank disclosure to the patient when it is discovered that poor quality care has been delivered or when there has been medical or hospital malpractice.

2 *Economy of care* The public has a right to economical care and to hospital management that operates efficiently and eliminates waste, such as unnecessary services and duplicative and unsafe facilities.

3 *Consumer input and participation in the decision process* The public has a right to have its voice heard in the management, control and planning of hospitals, and in the case of community hospitals it should be assured of a board of directors that represents a broad cross-section of the community. It has a right to see the end of present boards dominated by bankers, accountants, lawyers and heavy donors. It has a right to boards that can and do represent and serve the entire community.

4 *Access to information and answers about treatment* The patient has a right to full information on his diagnosis, treatment, and prognosis in terms he can understand. This should include information about alternative treatments and possible complications. The patient is entitled to have his questions answered on any phase of his hospital and medical care.

The hospital should make it easy for patients to know who they are dealing with. Every member of the hospital staff should wear a name tag with his full name and job title.

5 *Personal dignity* The patient has a right to personal dignity at all times. Among others, this includes the right to be treated without discrimination based on race, color, religion, national origin, ability to pay or source of payment; the right to considerate and respectful care; and the right to privacy and confidentiality of personal records. Those not directly involved in the treatment should affirmatively disclose their purposes and obtain permission of the patient to be present.

6 *Control of one's body and life* The patient has the right to control his body and life. This includes the patient's right to refuse treatment to the extent permitted by law, to be informed of the medical consequences of his action, and to leave the hospital when he desires to do so.

7 *Action on complaints and problems* The patient has a right to redress of grievances in a reasonably efficient and timely fashion. This means the hospital should establish formal grievance procedures and appoint ombudsmen or patient advocates to be certain that problems are identified and remedied.

8 *Disclosure of data about hospital* The public has a right to full information about the finances and activities of the hospital. This should include general information about assets, expenses, costs, profits, charges, occupancy and the like. This also includes information about the board of directors of the hospitals, physicians on the hospital staff, and all of its rules and regulations, including those which apply to his conduct as a patient. Finally, it includes information about financial aid available from the hospital.

This information should be voluntarily and automatically disclosed.

9 *Disclosure of conflict of interest problems* The patient and public has the right to full disclosure of any hospital relationships that pose an immediate or potential conflict of interest.

This means that every for-profit hospital should have strict procedures for enforcing the American Medical Association's ethical rule which is as follows: "When a physician has an interest in or owns a for-profit hospital to which he sends his patients, he has an affirmative ethical obligation to disclose this fact to his patient." This is only one possible hospital conflict of interest among many. For example, doctors may own outside laboratories, nursing homes, x-ray facilities and other health service facilities.

10 *Access to information about stay and records of case* The patient has a right to full information about his stay, including information about his bill and access to his hospital records. This includes detailed information about his hospital bill, including itemized charges. This information should be readily available regardless of the patient's source of payment.

11 *Continuity of care* The patient has a right to continuity of care. This includes timely response to his needs and appropriate transfer to other facilities.

The American Hospital Association's Bill of Rights talks about reasonable continuity of care. It adds that the patient: "has the right to know in advance what appointment times and physicians are available and where. The patient has the right to expect that the hospital will provide a mechanism whereby he is informed by his physician or a delegate of the physician of the patient's continuing health care requirements following discharge.''

12 *Consumer advocacy*   The public has a right to expect a hospital to behave as a consumer advocate rather than as a business headquarters for doctors and hospital officials. The hospital should affirmatively and aggressively move to protect the patient and his interests rather than rubber-stamp the demands of doctors. The hospital should provide leadership in improving health care for the community.*

*H. Denenberg, *Citizens Bill of Hospital Rights: What the Patient and Public Can and Should Expect from Our Hospitals*, Harrisburg, Pa., Pennsylvania Insurance Department, April 1973.

Media Resources

ABC News
7 West 66th St.
New York, N.Y. 10023

American Journal of Nursing Company
   (film rentals)
c/o Association Sterling Films
600 Grand Ave.
Ridgefield, N.J. 02657

American Journal of Nursing Company
   (all other audiovisuals)
Educational Services Division
10 Columbus Circle
New York, N.Y. 10019

American Medical Association Film
   Library
535 North Dearborn St.
Chicago, Ill. 60610

Association Instructional Materials
866 Third Ave.
New York, N.Y. 10022

Audio Visual Department
Youville Hospital
1575 Cambridge St.
Cambridge, Mass. 02138

Bailey Film Association
2211 Michigan Ave.
Santa Monica, Calif. 90404

Behavioral Sciences Tape Library
485 Main St.
Fort Lee, N.J. 07024

Bureau of Audiovisual Instruction
P.O. Box 2093
Madison, Wisc. 53701

Canadian Broadcasting Corporation
Learning Systems
Box 500, Station A
Toronto, Ontario, Canada

Center for Cassette Studies
81100 Webb Ave.
North Hollywood, Calif. 91605

Center for Continuing Education
Cook County Hospital
Evanston, Ill. 60201

Center for Death Education and
    Research
1167 Social Science Building
Minneapolis, Minn. 55455

Charles Eames Office
901 Washington St.
Venice, Calif. 90291

Church Films
2923 North Monroe St.
Spokane, Wash. 99205

Churchill Films
622 North Robertson Blvd.
Los Angeles, Calif. 90069

Concept Media
Box 2038, 1500 Adams Ave.
Costa Mesa, Calif. 92626

Contemporary Film–McGraw-Hill
Princeton Rd.
Hightstown, N.J. 18520

Creative Christian Communication
1855 South Shore Blvd.
Lake Oswego, Ore. 97304

Creative Resources
Box 1970
Waco, Tex.

Dawn Bible Students TV
611 Newton St.
San Francisco, Calif. 91340

Department of Medical Illustration
Division of Continuing Education
Medical College of South Carolina
80 Barre St.
Charlestown, S.C. 29401

Eccentric Circle Cinema Workshop

P.O. Box 1481   347 Florence Ave.
Evanston, Ill. 60204   Evanston, Ill. 60202

Film-Makers Library, Inc.
290 West End Ave.
New York, N.Y. 10023

Film Rental Library
The Espousal Center
554 Lexington St.
Waltham, Mass. 02154

Films, Inc.
1144 Wilmette Ave.
Wilmette, Ill. 60091

Foundation of Thanatology
67 Park Ave., Room 11-B
New York, N.Y. 10016

Franciscan Communication Center
12295 Santee St.
Los Angeles, Calif. 90015

Georgia Regional Medical Group
P. O. Box 26121
Atlanta, Ga. 30303

Gospel Films, Inc.
Box 455
Muskegon, Mich. 49443

Health Services Learning Resources
    Center
T-252 Health Sciences Building
University of Washington
Seattle, Wash. 98195

Indiana University
Audio-Visual Center
Bloomington, Ind. 47401

Inland Empire Human Resources Center
2 West Olive Ave.
Redlands, Calif. 92373

Macmillan Films, Inc.
34 Mac Questan Parkway South
Mount Vernon, N.Y. 10550

Mass Media
1720 Chauteau Ave.
St. Louis, Mo. 63103

Medical Education Resources Program
Indiana School of Medicine
1100 West Michigan St.
Indianapolis, Ind. 46202

Medical Media Network
10995 La Conte Ave.—Room 514
Los Angeles, Calif. 90024

Medical Resources Branch NMAC
   Annex
Station K
Atlanta, Ga. 30324

Mental Health Training Film Program
33 Fenwood Rd.
Boston, Mass. 02115

Milwaukee Regional Medical
   Instructional Television Station, Inc.
5000 West National Ave.
Milwaukee, Wisc. 53193

National Foundation for Sudden Infant
   Death
1501 Broadway
New York, N.Y. 10036

National Institutes of Mental Health
National Audiovisual Center, GSA
Washington, D.C. 20409

NBC Educational Enterprises
30 Rockefeller Plaza
New York, N.Y. 10020

Nebraska TV Council for Nursing
   Education
1800 North 33rd
Lincoln, Neb. 68503

Network for Continuing Medical
   Education
15 Columbus Circle
New York, N.Y. 10023

Oregon Division of Continuing Education
Film Library
P.O. Box 1491
Portland, Ore. 97201

Professional Research, Inc.
660 South Bonnie Brae St.
Los Angeles, Calif. 90057

Public Television Library
475 L'Enfant Plaza S.W.
Washington, D.C. 20024

Pyramid Films
Box 1048
Santa Monica, Calif. 90406

Roche Laboratories
Nutley, N.J. 07010

Ross Medical Association
1825 Sylvan Court
Flossmorr, Ill. 60422

Royal College of General Practitioners
Medical Recording Service Foundation
Kitts Craft, Writtle, Chelmsford
CMI 3 EH
England

Sunburst Communications
Pound Ridge, N.Y. 10576

Time/Life Films
Time/Life Building
43 West 16th St.
New York, N.Y. 10011

Train-Aide Educational Systems
229 North Central Ave.
Glendale, Calif. 91202

Trainex Corporation
P.O. Box 116
Garden Grove, Calif. 02642

TV Division
Naval Medical Training Institute
National Naval Medical Center
Bethesda, Md. 20014

University of California, Davis School of
   Medicine
Medical Learning Resources
Davis, Calif. 95616

University of California Extension Media
   Center
Berkeley, Calif. 94720

University of Iowa
Iowa City, Iowa 52240

University of Michigan AV Center
910 Maynard St.
Ann Arbor, Mich. 48104

University of Pittsburgh
School of Nursing
Pittsburgh, Pa. 15213

University of Southern California
Division of Research and Training in
  Rehabilitation
1739 Griffin Ave.
Los Angeles, Calif. 90031

University of Wisconsin
School of Nursing
Box 413
Milwaukee, Wisc. 53201

Walter Reed Army Medical Center
Video Tape Library—Room 1077
Building 34
Washington, D.C. 20305

WKYC-TV
1403 East Sixth St.
Cleveland, Ohio

Wombat Productions, Inc.
77 Tarrytown Rd.
White Plains, N.Y. 10607

Index